MASLD DIET COOKBOOK

1000+ DAYS OF EASY AND NUTRITIOUS RECIPES TO DETOXIFY, REJUVENATE YOUR LIVER AND PROMOTE LONGEVITY

KAREN EDMONDS

INTRODUCTION

Warmly welcome to the MASLD Diet Cookbook, an experience to improve your liver health with tasty and nutritious meals. Let me tell you what inspired this cookbook and why it is so essential.

Consider yourself exhausted, dealing with weight gain, and being diagnosed with Metabolic Dysfunction-Associated Steatotic Liver Disease (MASLD). This was my reality, and like many others battling liver health issues, I sought a means to recover energy via food.

The MASLD Diet is a lifestyle strategy that promotes liver function and overall metabolic health. I found a way to be healthier by focusing on nutrient-dense meals and limiting sweets and bad fats.

This cookbook is a treasure trove of liver-loving recipes that are both healthful and tasty. From filling breakfasts like the MASLD Breakfast Smoothie to hearty dinners like Baked lime and chilli Chicken, every meal is made using MASLD-friendly ingredients.

However, this cookbook is more than just a compilation of recipes; it is a guide to changing your relationship with food for improved health. Whether you are dealing with MASLD or simply want to improve the health of your liver, these dishes provide a tasty solution.

Join me in embracing the MASLD diet. Let is nurture our bodies and improve our health one tasty meal at a time. Here is to eating foods that love our livers back!

This introduction sets the tone for your MASLD Diet Cookbook, allowing readers to discover the transforming potential of food in promoting liver health and general well-being.

BE HAPPY AND STAY HEALTHY

CHAPTER 1: UNDERSTANDING METABOLIC DYSFUNCTION–ASSOCIATED STEATOTIC LIVER DISEASE (MASLD)

Metabolic Dysfunction-Associated Steatotic Liver Disease (MASLD), formerly known as Non-Alcoholic Fatty Liver Disease (NAFLD), is a disorder in which fat accumulates in the liver (hepatic steatosis) as a result of metabolic dysregulation. MASLD comprises a wide range of liver disorders, from basic fatty liver (steatosis) to non-alcoholic steatohepatitis (NASH), which causes inflammation and liver cell destruction. This condition is linked to metabolic diseases such obesity, insulin resistance, type 2 diabetes, dyslipidemia (abnormal lipid levels), and metabolic syndrome.

MASLD development is impacted by a variety of variables, including genetics, lifestyle, and food. One major contributor of MASLD is an excessive calorie intake, particularly from sweets and bad fats. These dietary components can cause fat to accumulate in the liver and aggravate inflammation, worsening the disease over time.

Key features of MASLD:

Steatosis (Fatty Liver): The main feature of MASLD is the excessive buildup of fat (triglycerides) inside liver cells. This can compromise liver function and promote inflammation and oxidative stress.

Inflammation: Fat accumulation can cause inflammation in the liver (non-alcoholic steatohepatitis, or NASH), resulting in liver cell damage and possible scarring (fibrosis).

Insulin Resistance: MASLD is significantly linked to insulin resistance, which occurs when cells become less receptive to insulin, resulting in elevated blood sugar levels. Insulin resistance increases fat storage in the liver.

Risk Factors: Obesity (particularly abdominal obesity), sedentary lifestyle, poor diet (rich in carbohydrates and saturated fats), type 2 diabetes, dyslipidemia, and metabolic syndrome are all known risk factors for MASLD.

What is MASLD?

The term MASLD refers to fatty liver disease in the context of metabolic dysfunction, emphasising the strong link between liver fat build-up and metabolic abnormalities. Unlike alcoholic fatty liver disease, MASLD develops in people who drink little or no alcohol.

How Diet Affects MASLD

Diet plays an important influence in the development and evolution of MASLD. Certain dietary components can cause fat build-up in the liver and worsen metabolic dysfunction, whilst others can assist relieve symptoms and enhance liver health. Here is how the diet affects MASLD:

Excessive Caloric Intake: Consuming more calories than the body requires, particularly from sweets and refined carbs, can cause excessive fat deposition in the liver.

Unhealthy Fats: A diet heavy in saturated and trans fats has been related to increased liver fat and inflammation. Limiting your consumption of these fats is essential for treating MASLD.

Added sweets: A high consumption of fructose and other sweets can lead to liver fat formation and insulin resistance. Avoiding sugary drinks and processed meals can be advantageous.

Nutrient-Dense Foods: Consuming a diet high in vegetables, fruits, whole grains, lean proteins (such as chicken, fish, and lentils), and healthy fats (such as olive oil and nuts) will help decrease liver fat and enhance metabolic health.

Weight Management: Achieving and maintaining a healthy weight via nutrition and exercise is essential for treating MASLD. Even small weight loss can result in considerable benefits in liver function.

Balanced Macronutrients: A diet rich in protein, healthy fats, and complex carbs can help manage blood sugar levels and improve liver function.

Understanding MASLD entails recognising its link to metabolic illnesses as well as the effect of nutrition on liver function. A healthy, balanced diet based on nutrient-dense foods and weight control is critical for avoiding and treating MASLD.

CHAPTER 2: OVERVIEW OF THE MASLD DIET PRINCIPLES

The MASLD Diet is a dietary strategy designed to improve liver health and metabolic function in those who have metabolic dysfunction-associated fatty liver disease (MASLD). The MASLD Diet promotes nutrient-dense, whole foods while avoiding sugar, harmful fats, and processed foods.

Key Ingredients of the MASLD Diet:

High-Fiber Foods: A range of fiber-rich foods, including vegetables, fruits, whole grains, legumes, and nuts, are recommended. Fibre helps to manage blood sugar levels, increases fullness, and improves intestinal health.

Healthy Fats: The MASLD Diet emphasises the importance of eating healthy fats including avocados, nuts, seeds, and olive oil. These fats are rich in important fatty acids and have anti-inflammatory characteristics that promote liver function.

Lean Proteins: Consuming lean protein sources such as poultry, fish, tofu, and lentils aids to support muscle mass and metabolism while avoiding extra saturated fat.

Limiting Added Sugars: Reducing your consumption of added sugars and sugary beverages is critical for lowering liver fat and boosting insulin sensitivity.

Reducing Saturated and Trans Fats: Limiting saturated fats in fatty cuts of meat, full-fat dairy products, and processed meals, as well as avoiding trans fats in partly hydrogenated oils, is critical for liver function.

Moderate Alcohol drinking: Individuals with MASLD should restrict or avoid alcohol drinking totally since it might harm the liver even more.

Portion Control and Balanced Meals: Practicing portion control and eating balanced meals rich in a range of nutrients (protein, carbs, fats, and fibre) helps to keep blood sugar levels constant and promotes overall metabolic health.

Benefits of the MASLD Diet for Liver Health:

Reduces Liver Fat: The MASLD Diet focuses on foods that promote liver fat loss, which leads to better liver function and a lower risk of inflammation and fibrosis.

Improves Insulin Sensitivity: By emphasising whole foods and limiting sweets, the MASLD Diet helps to enhance insulin sensitivity, which is useful for those who suffer from insulin resistance and type 2 diabetes, both of which are frequent in MASLD.

Supports Weight Management: Adopting the MASLD Diet can help with weight control, which is vital for lowering liver fat formation and improving metabolic parameters.

Anti-inflammatory Effects: The MASLD Diet, which is high in antioxidants and anti-inflammatory elements, helps to lower systemic inflammation, which is good for your liver and general health.

Promotes Overall Metabolic Health: Following the MASLD Diet principles improves overall metabolic health, including lipid metabolism, blood sugar management, and cardiovascular health, all of which are directly related to MASLD.

The MASLD Diet is a dietary strategy that promotes liver health and metabolic function through balanced nutrition, emphasising nutrient-dense foods while minimising sweets and harmful fats. Following the MASLD Diet principles can result in considerable improvements in liver function, insulin sensitivity, and general metabolic well-being in those with MASLD. It is suggested that you consult with a healthcare physician or certified dietitian to customise the MASLD Diet for your specific requirements and health objectives.

CHAPTER 3: BREAKFAST RECIPES

Creamy Almond Butter Porridge

Ingredients:

- 1/2 cup of rolled oats
- 1 cup of almond milk (or any milk of your choice)
- 1 tablespoon of almond butter
- 1 tablespoon of maple syrup or honey (optional, for sweetness)
- 1/2 teaspoon of vanilla extract
- Pinch of salt
- Toppings of your choice (e.g., sliced bananas, berries, chopped nuts, or seeds)

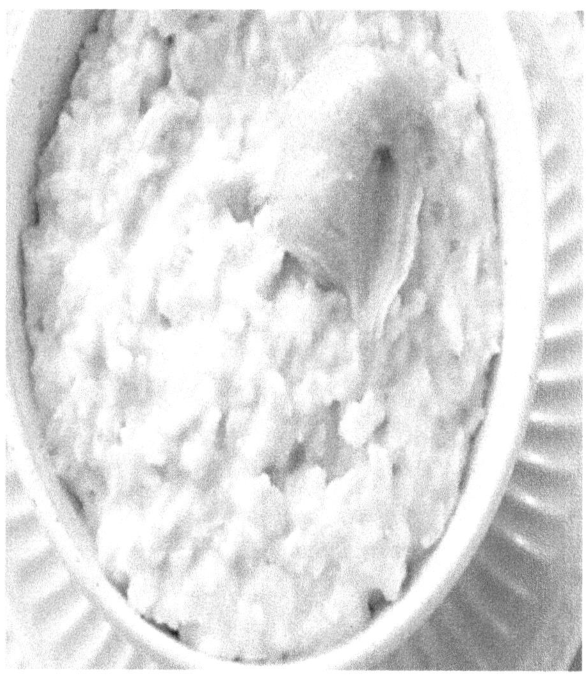

Preparation:

- In a small saucepan, cook the rolled oats and almond milk over medium heat.
- Combine the almond butter, maple syrup or honey (if using), vanilla essence, and a sprinkle of salt.
- Cook the mixture, stirring regularly, until the oats are cooked and the porridge achieves the desired consistency (5-7 minutes). To achieve a creamier texture, add extra milk as needed.
- After cooking, take the porridge from the heat and let it sit for a minute to thicken.
- Place the porridge in a bowl and top with your preferred toppings, such as sliced bananas, berries, chopped almonds, or seeds

Nutritional Value (Approximate per Serving):

Calories: 300-350 kcal

Protein: 8-10 grams

Fat: 12-15 grams (mainly from healthy fats in almond butter)

Carbohydrates: 40-45 grams

Fibre: 5-7 grams

Sugar: 8-12 grams (depending on sweetness added)

Calcium: 200-250 mg (from almond milk)

Iron: 2-3 mg (from oats and almond butter)

Notes

Your

Observation

Gluten-Free Breakfast Pancakes

Ingredients:

- 2 eggs
- 1/2 cup of cottage cheese
- 1/2 cup of gluten-free oats
- 6 olives, sliced
- 1/2 teaspoon of dried oregano
- Salt and pepper, to taste
- Olive oil or other cooking oil for frying

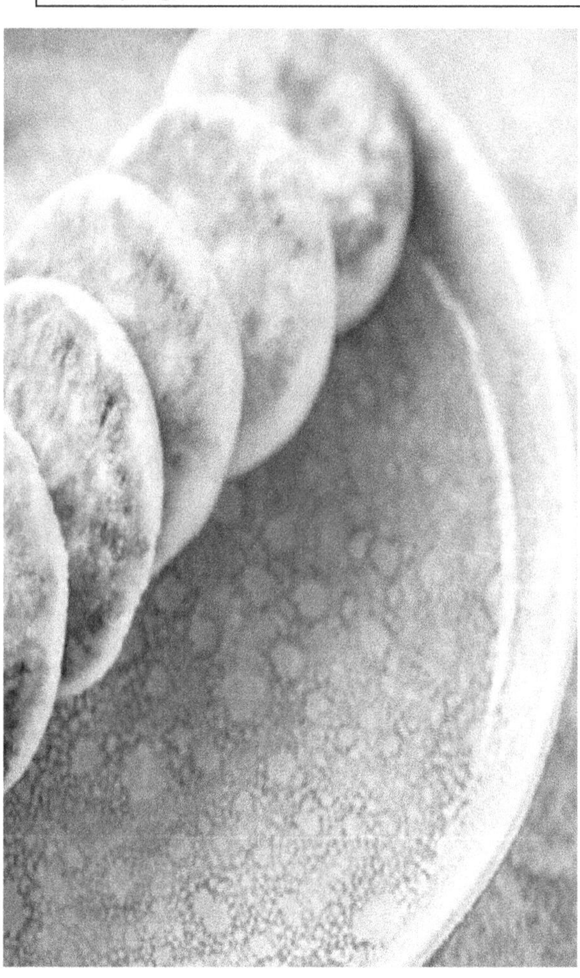

Preparations:

- In a blender or food processor, add together the eggs, cottage cheese, gluten-free oats, dried oregano, salt, and pepper.
- Blend until smooth and thoroughly incorporated. The oats will help bind the pancake mixture and serve as a gluten-free substitute to flour.
- Stir the sliced olives into the pancake batter. You may also save some olives to decorate the pancakes afterward.
- Heat a non-stick skillet or frying pan over medium heat, then add a tiny quantity of olive or cooking oil.
- Pour a dollop of the pancake batter onto the skillet, roughly 1/4 cup each pancake. Using the back of a spoon, spread the batter into a spherical shape if necessary.
- Cook the pancakes for 2-3 minutes on one side, or until golden brown and firm around the edges.
- Flip the pancakes carefully and cook for another 1-2 minutes on the other side, until cooked through and lightly browned.
- Repeat with the remaining batter, adding additional oil to the skillet as necessary between batches.
- Serve the gluten-free savoury pancakes warm, garnished with extra sliced olives as desired.

Nutritional value (Approximate per Serving, based on 2 servings):

Calories: 250-300 kcal

Protein: 16-18 grams

Fat: 14-16 grams

Carbohydrates: 16-18 grams

Fibre: 2-3 grams

Sugar: 2-3 grams

Notes

Your

Observation

Gluten Free Cinnamon Rice Porridge

Ingredients:

- 1 cup of cooked rice (white or brown rice works well)
- 1 1/4 cups of milk of your choice (almond milk, coconut milk, or dairy milk)
- 4 Medjool dates, pitted and chopped
- 1/4 teaspoon of ground cinnamon
- 1 teaspoon of Nature Sweet natural sugar alternative (or sweetener of your choice)
- Fresh fruit (such as sliced bananas, berries, or apples) and nuts (such as chopped almonds or walnuts) for serving

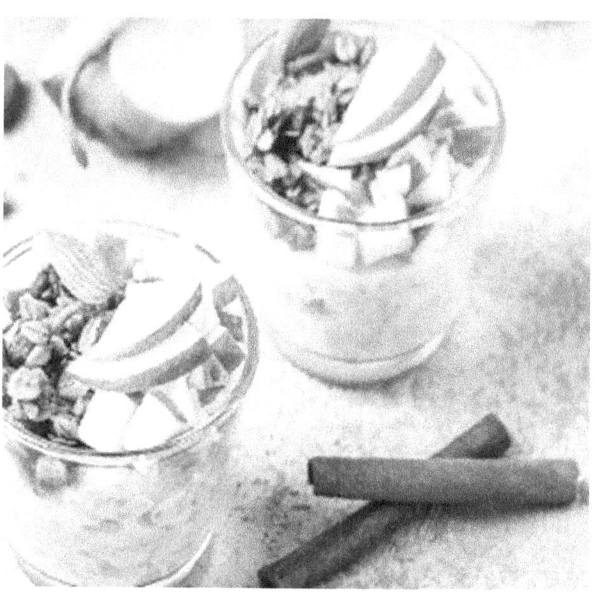

Preparations:

- In a small saucepan, mix together the cooked rice, milk, chopped Medjool dates, crushed cinnamon, and Nature Sweet natural sugar replacement.
- Place the saucepan over medium heat and bring to a simmer, stirring regularly.
- Once simmering, decrease the heat to low and cook for 5-7 minutes, or until the mixture reaches the desired porridge consistency. Stir occasionally to avoid sticking.
- Taste the porridge and adjust the sweetness as needed by adding additional sugar substitute.
- Remove the pot from the heat and allow the porridge to cool for a minute.
- Serve the gluten-free cinnamon rice porridge warm in bowls.
- To add texture and flavour, top each dish with fresh fruit slices and chopped almonds.
- Enjoy your tasty and nutritious gluten-free cinnamon rice porridge as a hearty breakfast or snack!

Nutritional value:

Calories: Approximately 280-320 kcal

Protein: 5-7 grams

Fat: 4-6 grams

Carbohydrates: 60-65 grams

Dietary Fibre: 3-5 grams

Sugars: 30-35 grams (naturally occurring from dates and rice)

Calcium: 200-250 mg (from milk)

Iron: 1-2 mg

Potassium: 300-400 mg

Notes

Your

Observation

Low Carb Breakfast Eggs

Ingredients:

- 1 cup of chopped pumpkin pieces
- 8 eggs
- 1/4 cup of canned full-fat coconut milk
- 2 tablespoons of olive oil, or animal fat (such as bacon fat)
- 2 tablespoons of chopped olives
- 1 teaspoon of dried oregano
- 1 teaspoon of ground cumin
- Salt and pepper, to taste
- Chopped spinach (optional)

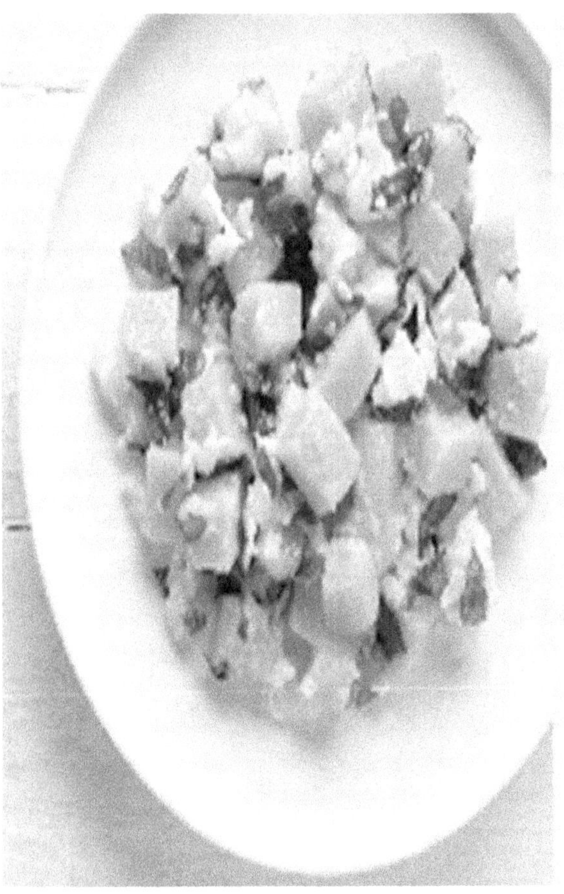

Preparations:

- Preheat the oven to 400 °F (200 °C).
- Steam the chopped pumpkin in a microwave-safe dish with a little water for 3-4 minutes, or until soft. Alternatively, bake the pumpkin slices in the oven until soft and faintly caramelised.
- In a mixing dish, crack the eggs and whisk them with the canned coconut milk until thoroughly blended.
- Heat the olive oil, ghee, or animal fat in a large oven-safe pan over medium heat.
- Sauté the cooked pumpkin chunks in the skillet for 2-3 minutes, or until they begin to colour slightly.
- Cook for another minute, stirring in the chopped olives, dry oregano, and powdered cumin to unleash the flavours.
- If using chopped spinach, toss it into the pan and heat until wilted.
- Pour the egg and coconut milk mixture into the skillet with the vegetables.
- Season with salt and pepper to taste.
- Allow the mixture to simmer undisturbed on the hob for about 2-3 minutes, or until the edges begin to harden.
- Place the pan in the preheated oven for 12-15 minutes, or until the eggs are completely set and cooked through.
- Remove from the oven and allow it cool slightly before slicing and serving.

> - Optional: To complete the meal, serve the low-carb breakfast eggs with a side salad or avocado slices.

Nutritional Value (Approximate per Serving):

Calories: Approximately 300-350 kcal

Protein: 16-18 grams

Fat: 22-24 grams

Saturated Fat: 9-11 grams

Carbohydrates: 8-10 grams

Dietary Fibre: 2-3 grams

Sugars: 3-4 grams

Sodium: 400-500 mg

Notes

Your

Observation

CHAPTER 4: LUNCH RECIPES

Pumpkin and Walnut Salad

Ingredients:

- 2 cups of diced pumpkin (about 1-inch cubes)
- 1 tablespoon of olive oil
- Salt and pepper, to taste
- 4 cups of mixed salad greens (such as spinach, arugula, or mixed baby greens)
- 1/2 cup of walnut halves
- 1/4 cup of crumbled feta cheese (optional)
- Balsamic vinaigrette dressing

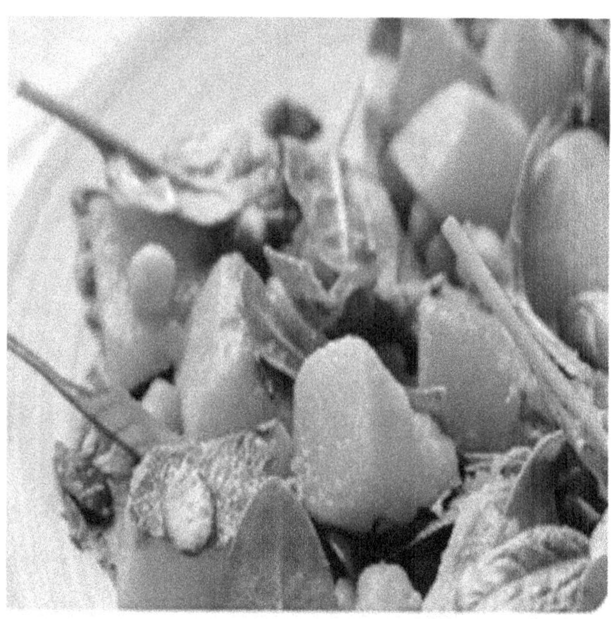

Preparations:

- Preheat the oven to 400 °F (200 °C).
- Put the chopped pumpkin on a baking sheet. Drizzle with olive oil, then season with salt and pepper. Toss to coat evenly.
- Roast the pumpkin in a warm oven for 20-25 minutes, or until soft and slightly caramelised. Remove from the oven and allow it cool slightly.
- In a dry skillet over medium heat, toast the walnut halves for 3-5 minutes, tossing regularly, until gently browned and aromatic. Take cautious not to burn them. Remove from heat and allow to cool.
- In a large salad dish, add the mixed greens, roasted pumpkin cubes, and toasted walnut halves.
- If using, add crumbled feta cheese over the salad.
- Drizzle the salad with balsamic vinaigrette dressing, starting with a few teaspoons and adding more to taste. Gently toss everything to provide a uniform coating.
- Serve the pumpkin and walnut salad immediately as a side or main course.

Nutritional Value (Approximate per Serving):

Calories: Approximately 250-300 kcal

Protein: 5-7 grams

Fat: 20-25 grams

Saturated Fat: 2-3 grams

Carbohydrates: 15-20 grams

Dietary Fibre: 4-6 grams

Sugars: 5-8 grams

Sodium: 200-300 mg

Notes

Your

Observation

Shrimp And Broccoli Stir Fry

Ingredients:

- 1 pound of big shrimp, peeled and deveined
- 3 cups of broccoli florets
- 2 tablespoons of soy sauce (use tamari for gluten-free option)
- 1 tablespoon of oyster sauce (optional)
- 1 tablespoon of hoisin sauce (optional)
- 2 cloves of minced garlic
- 1-inch piece of ginger, grated
- 2 tablespoons of vegetable oil (such as canola or peanut oil)
- Salt and pepper, to taste
- Cooked rice or noodles, for serving

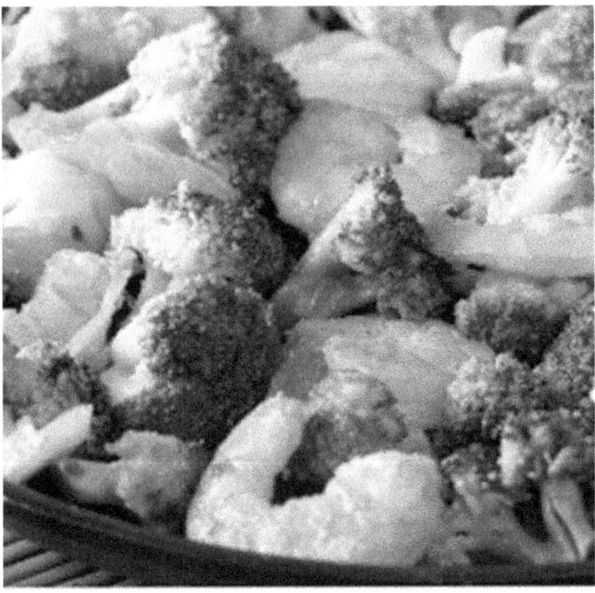

Preparations:

- Add together the soy sauce, oyster sauce (if using), and hoisin sauce in a small bowl. Put aside.
- Heat 1 tablespoon vegetable oil in a large pan over medium-high heat.
- Season the prawns in the pan with salt and pepper. Cook the prawns for 2-3 minutes, stirring periodically, until they are pink and opaque. Remove the prawns from the skillet and set it aside.
- In the same skillet, add the remaining tablespoon of oil. Stir in the minced garlic and grated ginger, cooking for about 30 seconds or until fragrant.
- Stir-fry the broccoli florets in the pan for 3-4 minutes, or until tender and crisp.
- Return the cooked prawns to the skillet.
- Pour the sauce (soy, oyster and hoisin sauce) over the prawns and broccoli. Stir carefully to uniformly coat everything, then cook for a further 1-2 minutes until well cooked.
- Taste and adjust seasoning with salt and pepper as required.
- Serve the prawns and broccoli stir-fry hot with prepared rice or noodles

Nutritional Value (Approximate per Serving, excluding rice/noodles):

Calories: Approximately 250-300 kcal

Protein: 30-35 grams

Fat: 10-12 grams

Saturated Fat: 1-2 grams

Carbohydrates: 10-12 grams

Dietary Fibre: 3-4 grams

Sugars: 2-3 grams

Sodium: 800-1000 mg (depending on sauce used)

Your

Observation

Sugar-Free Beef Ginger Stir Fry

Ingredients:

- 1 pound beef sirloin or flank steak, thinly sliced against the grain
- 2 tablespoons of soy sauce (use tamari for gluten-free option)
- 1 tablespoon of rice vinegar
- 1 tablespoon of sesame oil
- 2 tablespoons of olive oil or vegetable oil, divided
- 3 cloves of minced garlic
- 1 tablespoon of fresh ginger, minced
- 1 bell pepper, sliced
- 1 onion, sliced
- 2 cups of broccoli florets
- Salt and pepper, to taste
- Optional garnish: sliced green onions and sesame seeds

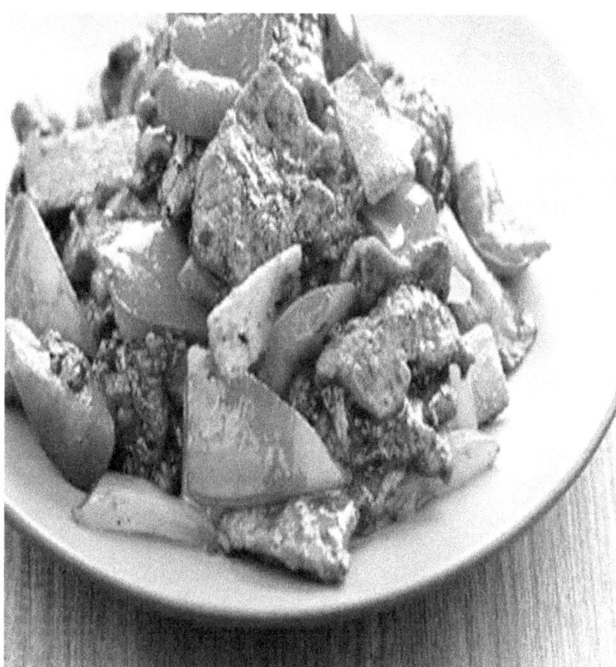

Preparations:

- Marinate the sliced beef in a basin with soy sauce, rice vinegar, and sesame oil. Set aside for at least 15-20 minutes.
- Heat 1 tablespoon olive oil in a large pan or wok over medium-high heat.
- Add the minced garlic and ginger to the pan and cook for about 30 seconds, or until fragrant.
- Add the marinated meat to the pan in one layer. Cook for 2-3 minutes, without stirring, until the meat is seared and browned on one side. Then, stir-fry for a further 2-3 minutes, or until the meat is cooked to your liking. Remove the steak from the skillet and put it aside.
- In the same skillet, heat the last tablespoon of olive oil.
- Add the sliced bell pepper, onion, and broccoli florets to the skillet. Stir-fry the veggies for about 4-5 minutes, or until they are soft and crisp.
- Return the cooked meat to the pan and add the veggies. Stir everything up until combined.
- Season the stir-fry with salt and pepper, to taste.
- Cook for another 1-2 minutes to ensure everything is thoroughly heated.
- Optional: Before serving, sprinkle sliced green onions and sesame seeds over the beef ginger stir-fry.
- Serve the sugar-free beef ginger stir-fry hot, with cooked rice or cauliflower rice.

Nutritional Value (Approximate per Serving, excluding rice):

Calories: Approximately 300-350 kcal

Protein: 25-30 grams

Fat: 20-25 grams

Saturated Fat: 5-7 grams

Carbohydrates: 10-12 grams

Dietary Fibre: 3-4 grams

Sugars: 4-6 grams (naturally occurring from vegetables)

Sodium: 600-700 mg (depending on soy sauce used)

Notes

Your

Observation

Immune Boosting Garlic Pesto

Ingredients:

- 2 cups of fresh basil leaves, packed
- 3 cloves of garlic, peeled
- 1/2 cup of pine nuts or walnuts, toasted
- 1/2 cup of grated Parmesan cheese (optional, omit for dairy-free version)
- 1/2 cup of extra-virgin olive oil
- 1 lemon, juiced
- Salt and pepper, to taste

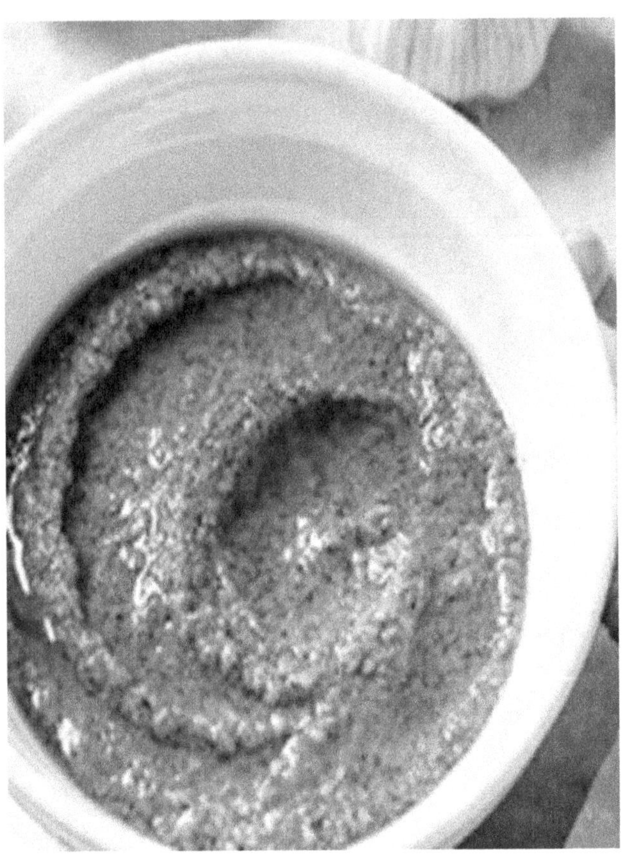

Preparations:

- Mix basil leaves, peeled garlic cloves, and roasted pine nuts (or walnuts) in a food processor or blender.
- Pulse the items until they are finely minced and well blended.
- Add the grated Parmesan cheese (if using) and pulse again to combine.
- With the food processor running, carefully sprinkle in the extra-virgin olive oil until the pesto is smooth and creamy.
- Add lemon juice, salt, and pepper to taste. Blend again until everything is well blended.
- Taste the garlic pesto and adjust seasoning as required, adding more salt, pepper, or lemon juice to your liking.
- *Storage:*
- Transfer the garlic pesto to a well sealed container or jar.
- To prevent oxidation, sprinkle a thin coating of olive oil over the pesto before closing.
- Refrigerate for up to a week, or freeze in ice cube trays for extended storage.
- *Ways to Eat Immune-Boosting Garlic Pesto:*
- Toss with cooked pasta to make a fast and tasty pasta meal.
- Spread on sandwiches or wraps for a tasty condiment.
- Serve as a topping on grilled chicken, fish, or vegetables.
- Mix into soups or stews to enhance the flavour.

- Spread on toasted bread or crackers for an easy appetiser.

Nutritional Information (Approximate per Serving):

Calories: Approximately 150-200 kcal (per 2 tablespoon serving)

Protein: 3-5 grams

Fat: 15-20 grams

Saturated Fat: 2-3 grams

Carbohydrates: 2-4 grams

Fibre: 1-2 grams

Sugars: 0 grams

Sodium: 100-150 mg (depending on salt added)

Notes

Your

Observation

CHAPTER 5: DINNER RECIPES

Baked Lime And Chilli Chicken

Ingredients:

- 4 boneless, skinless chicken breasts
- 2 limes, juiced
- Zest of 1 lime
- 2 tablespoons of olive oil
- 2 cloves of minced garlic
- 1 teaspoon of chili powder (adjust to taste)
- 1/2 teaspoon of paprika
- 1/2 teaspoon of cumin
- Salt and pepper, to taste
- Fresh cilantro or parsley, chopped (for garnish)

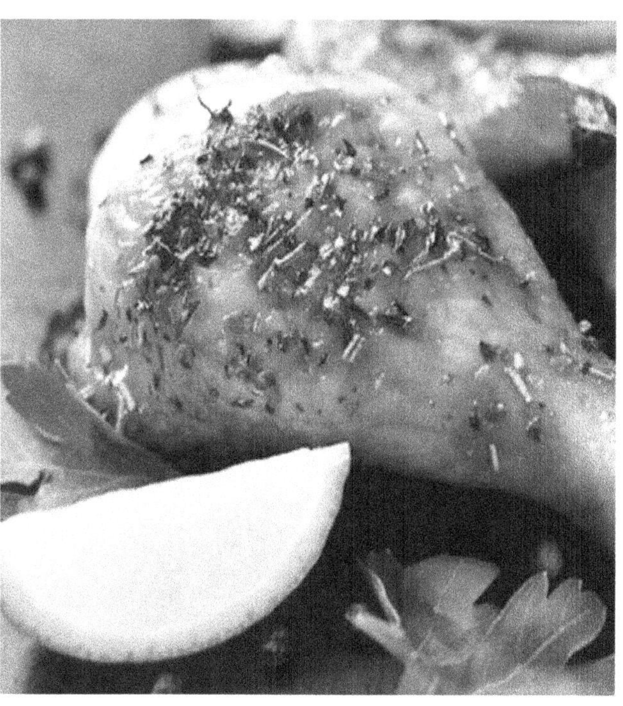

Preparations:

- Preheat the oven to 400°F (200°C), and gently butter a baking dish.
- In a mixing bowl, combine the lime juice, zest, olive oil, chopped garlic, chilli powder, paprika, cumin, salt, and pepper. Mix well to make a marinade.
- Place the chicken breasts in a baking dish and pour the marinade over them, making sure they are uniformly covered.
- Allow the chicken to marinade for 20-30 minutes (or longer in the refrigerator for more flavour).
- Bake the chicken in the preheated oven for 20-25 minutes, or until it is well cooked and has reached an internal temperature of 165°F (75°C).
- If desired, broil the chicken for an additional 2-3 minutes to get a golden brown top.
- Remove the baked lime and chilli chicken from the oven and set aside for a few minutes.
- Garnish with chopped fresh cilantro or parsley before serving.
- *Serve:*
- Serve the baked lime and chilli chicken with rice, quinoa, or any salad of your choosing.
- Drizzle the leftover pan juices over the chicken to add flavour.

Nutritional Information (Approximate per Serving):

Calories: Approximately 250-300 kcal (per chicken breast)

Protein: 25-30 grams

Fat: 12-15 grams

Saturated Fat: 2-3 grams

Carbohydrates: 5-8 grams

Fiber: 1-2 grams

Sugars: 1-2 grams

Sodium: 400-500 mg

Notes

Your

Observation

Low Carb Lamb Stew

Ingredients:

- 1.5 pounds boneless lamb stew meat, chpped into cubes
- 2 tablespoons of olive oil
- 1 onion, diced
- 2 cloves of minced garlic
- 2 celery stalks, chopped
- 2 carrots, peeled and chopped (optional, omit for lower carb)
- 1 small turnip, peeled and diced
- 1 teaspoon of dried thyme
- 1 teaspoon of dried rosemary
- 1 bay leaf
- Salt and pepper, to taste
- 4 cups of beef or vegetable broth
- 1/2 cup of dry red wine (optional, omit for alcohol-free version)
- 1 cup of diced tomatoes (canned or fresh)
- 1 cup of chopped kale or spinach
- Chopped fresh parsley, for garnish

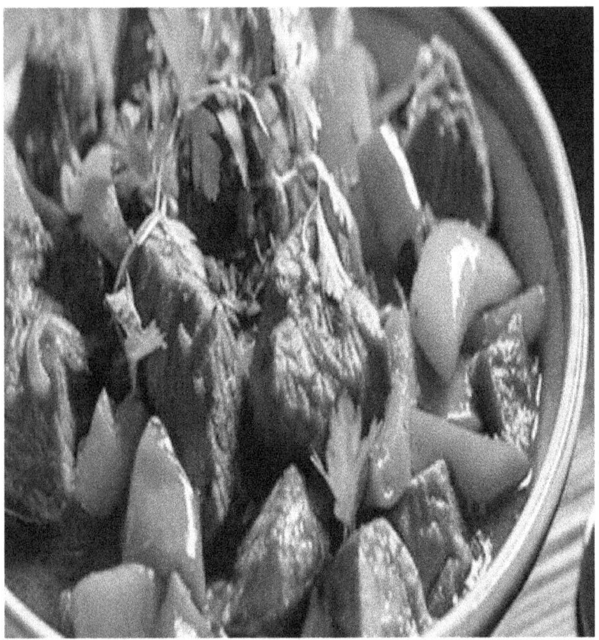

Preparations:

- Heat the olive oil in a big saucepan or Dutch oven over medium-high heat.
- Brown the chopped lamb stew meat on both sides, approximately 5-7 minutes. Remove the browned lamb from the saucepan and put it aside.
- In the same saucepan, combine the chopped onion, minced garlic, celery, carrots (if using), and turnip. Sauté the veggies for 5-6 minutes, until they begin to soften.
- Return the browned lamb to the pot. Combine the dried thyme, rosemary, bay leaf, salt, and pepper. Stir to mix.
- Pour in the beef or vegetable broth and red wine (if used), scraping away any browned pieces on the bottom of the saucepan.
- Add the chopped tomatoes to the saucepan and bring it to a simmer.
- Reduce the heat to low, cover the pot, and allow the stew simmer for 1.5 to 2 hours, or until the lamb is soft and well cooked. Stir occasionally.
- In the last 10 minutes of simmering, add the chopped kale or spinach to the stew. Stir until the greens have wilted.
- Taste the stew and season with more salt and pepper as needed.
- Remove the bay leaf before serving.
- Garnish the low carb lamb stew with fresh parsley and serve hot.

Nutritional Value(Approximate per Serving):

Calories: Approximately 350-400 kcal

Protein: 30-35 grams

Fat: 20-25 grams

Saturated Fat: 8-10 grams

Carbohydrates: 10-15 grams

Dietary Fiber: 3-5 grams

Sugars: 5-8 grams

Sodium: 800-1000 mg (depending on broth used)

Notes

Your

Observation

Roast Pumpkin And Cumin Hummus

Ingredients:

- 1 cup of cooked chickpeas (canned or cooked from dried)
- 1 cup of roasted pumpkin puree (see instructions below)
- 2 cloves of minced garlic
- 2 tablespoons of tahini (sesame seed paste)
- 1 lemon, juiced
- 1 teaspoon of ground cumin
- 1/2 teaspoon of smoked paprika (optional)
- Salt and pepper, to taste
- 2-4 tablespoons of olive oil
- Water, as needed

For Roasted Pumpkin Puree:

- 1 small pumpkin (about 2 pounds)
- 1-2 tablespoons of olive oil
- Salt and pepper, to taste

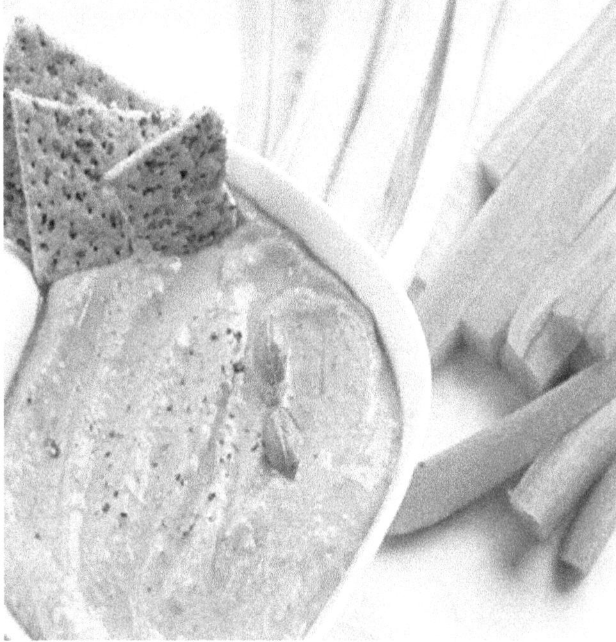

Preparations:

- *Roasting a Pumpkin:*
- Preheat the oven to 400 degrees Fahrenheit (200 degrees Celsius) and line a baking sheet with parchment paper.
- Cut the pumpkin in half, then scrape out the seeds and stringy pulp.
- Drizzle olive oil over the sliced edges of the pumpkin and season with salt and pepper.
- Place the pumpkin halves, cut side down, on the prepared baking sheet.
- Roast in a preheated oven for 40-50 minutes, or until the pumpkin flesh is fork soft and caramelised.
- Let the roasted pumpkin cool slightly before scooping out the meat and discarding the skin.
- For the hummus recipe, measure out 1 cup of roasted pumpkin flesh. Any leftover pumpkin puree can be saved for further applications.
- *Making Roasted Pumpkin and Cumin Hummus*:
- In a food processor, mix together the cooked chickpeas, roasted pumpkin puree, minced garlic, tahini, lemon juice, ground cumin, smoked paprika (if using), salt, and pepper.
- Process until smooth and well incorporated, scraping down the sides of the food processor as required.
- Drizzle 2 tablespoons olive oil into the food processor while it's running. Add extra olive oil as needed to get the desired consistency.

- If the hummus is too thick, add water a tablespoon at a time until it has a creamy consistency.
- Taste the hummus and add extra salt, pepper, or lemon juice if desired.
- Transfer the roasted pumpkin and cumin hummus to a serving dish.
- Drizzle with more olive oil and top with a pinch of ground cumin or smoky paprika.
- Hummus can be served with pita bread, crackers, fresh vegetables, or used as a spread in sandwiches or wraps

Nutritional Value (Approximate per Serving):

Calories: Approximately 150-200 kcal (per serving)

Protein: 4-6 grams

Fat: 8-10 grams

Saturated Fat: 1-2 grams

Carbohydrates: 15-20 grams

Dietary Fiber: 4-6 grams

Sugars: 2-3 grams

Sodium: 150-200 mg

Notes

Your

Observation

Raw Carrot And Almond Salad

Ingredients:

- 4 average carrots, peeled and grated
- 1/2 cup of slivered almonds
- 2 tablespoons of fresh lemon juice
- 2 tablespoons of extra-virgin olive oil
- 1 tablespoon of honey or maple syrup (optional, for sweetness)
- 1/4 teaspoon of ground cumin
- Salt and pepper, to taste
- Fresh parsley or cilantro, chopped (for garnish)

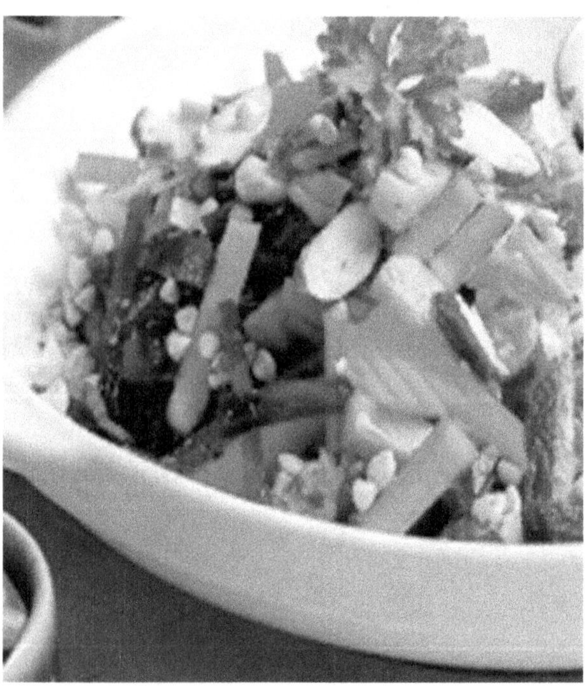

Preparations:

- In a large bowl, combine the grated carrots and slivered almonds.
- In a small bowl or jar, whisk together the fresh lemon juice, extra-virgin olive oil, honey or maple syrup (if using), ground cumin, salt, and pepper.
- Pour the dressing over the carrots and almonds. Toss well to coat everything evenly.
- Taste the salad and adjust seasoning with more salt, pepper, or lemon juice if needed.
- Let the carrot and almond salad sit for 10-15 minutes to allow the flavors to meld together.
- Before serving, garnish with chopped fresh parsley or cilantro.
- Optional Additions:
- Add a handful of raisins or dried cranberries for a touch of sweetness and chewiness.
- Include finely chopped red onion or scallions for added flavor and crunch.
- Toss in a handful of chopped fresh mint or basil leaves for a refreshing twist.

Nutritional value (Approximate per Serving):

Calories: Approximately 150-200 kcal

Protein: 3-5 grams

Fat: 10-12 grams

Saturated Fat: 1-2 grams

Carbohydrates: 15-20 grams

Dietary Fiber: 4-6 grams

Sugars: 8-10 grams

Sodium: 100-150 mg

Notes

Your

Observation

CHAPTER 6: SNACKS AND APPETIZERS

Chocolate Chia

Ingredients:

- 1/4 cup of chia seeds
- 1 cup of almond milk (or any milk of preference)
- 2 tablespoons of unsweetened cocoa powder
- 1-2 tablespoons of maple syrup or honey (adjust to taste)
- 1/2 teaspoon of vanilla extract
- Optional toppings: sliced strawberries, banana slices, chopped nuts, coconut flakes

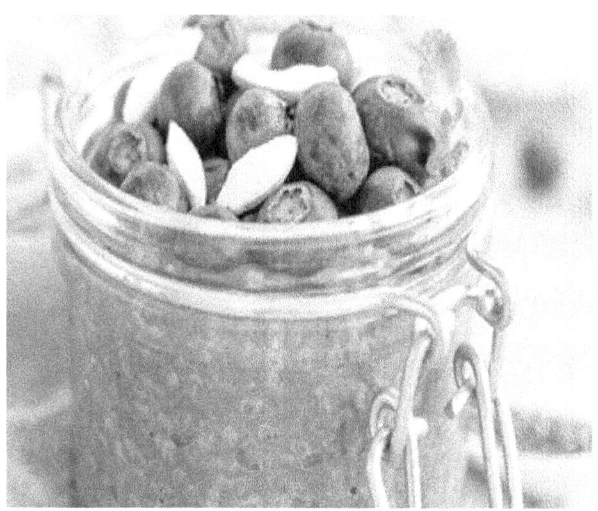

Preparations:

- In a mixing dish or container, add chia seeds, almond milk, unsweetened cocoa powder, maple syrup or honey, and vanilla extract.
- Whisk everything together until well blended.
- Cover the bowl or jar and chill for at least 2-3 hours, ideally overnight. To prevent clumping, stir or shake the mixture occasionally during the first hour.
- After chilling, the chia seeds absorb the liquid and thicken into a pudding-like consistency.
- If the custard is too thick for your palate, add a little extra almond milk to get the right texture.
- Divide the chocolate chia seed pudding across serving dishes or glasses.
- Add your favourite toppings, such as sliced strawberries, banana slices, chopped almonds, or coconut flakes.
- Serve cold and enjoy!

Nutritional value (Approximate per Serving):

Calories: Approximately 200-250 kcal

Protein: 6-8 grams

Fat: 10-12 grams

Saturated Fat: 1-2 grams

Carbohydrates: 25-30 grams

Dietary Fiber: 12-15 grams

Sugars: 10-15 grams

Sodium: 100-150 mg

Notes

Your

Observation

Sugar-Free Grilled Peaches Recipe

Ingredients:

- 4 ripe peaches, halved and pitted
- 1 tablespoon of olive oil or melted coconut oil
- Ground cinnamon, for sprinkling (optional)
- Fresh mint leaves, for garnish (optional)

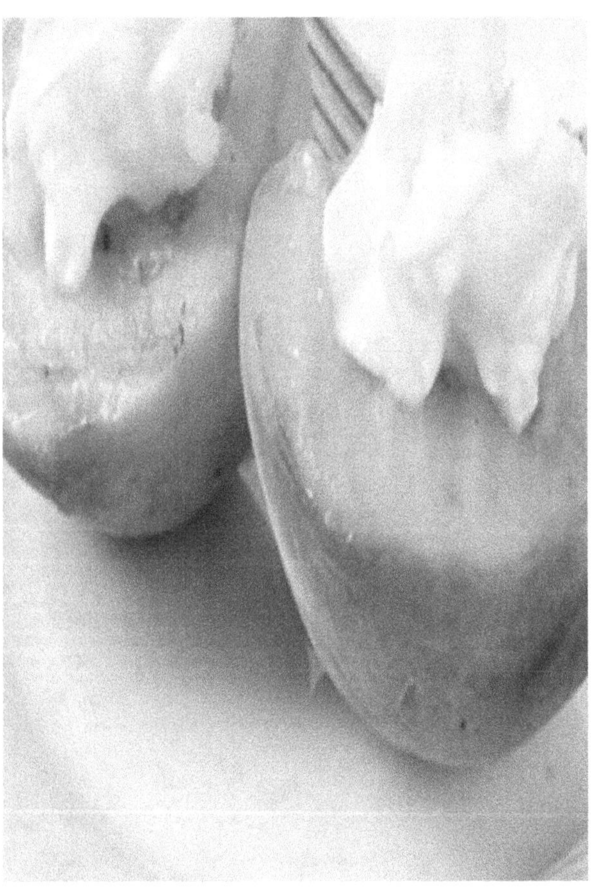

Preparations:

- Preheat the grill or grill pan to medium-high heat.
- While the grill is heated, prepare the peaches. Cut each peach in half to remove the pit.
- Brush the cut side of each peach half with olive oil or heated coconut oil to avoid sticking and encourage caramelization.
- Place the peach halves, cut side down, on the hot grill.
- Grill the peaches for 3-4 minutes each side, or until they have lovely grill marks and are tender yet firm.
- Optional: For extra flavour, sprinkle some ground cinnamon over the grilled peaches.
- Remove the cooked peaches from the grill and place them on a serving plate.
- Allow the peaches to cool slightly before serving.
- Garnish with fresh mint leaves, if preferred, to add colour and freshness.
- Serve sugar-free grilled peaches as a light and nutritious dessert or snack. You may eat them on their own or with a dollop of Greek yoghurt or a scoop of vanilla ice cream for an extra delight.

Nutritional value (Approximate per Serving):

Calories: Approximately 60-70 kcal per peach half

Fat: 2-3 grams

Carbohydrates: 10-12 grams

Fiber: 2-3 grams

Sugars: 8-10 grams (naturally occurring sugars in peaches)

Protein: 1 gram

Vitamin C: 7-9 mg

Notes

Your

Observation

Easy banana pancakes

Ingredients:

- 1 ripe banana
- 2 eggs
- 1/4 teaspoon of baking powder (optional, for fluffier pancakes)
- 1/2 teaspoon of vanilla extract (optional)
- Butter or oil, for greasing the pan

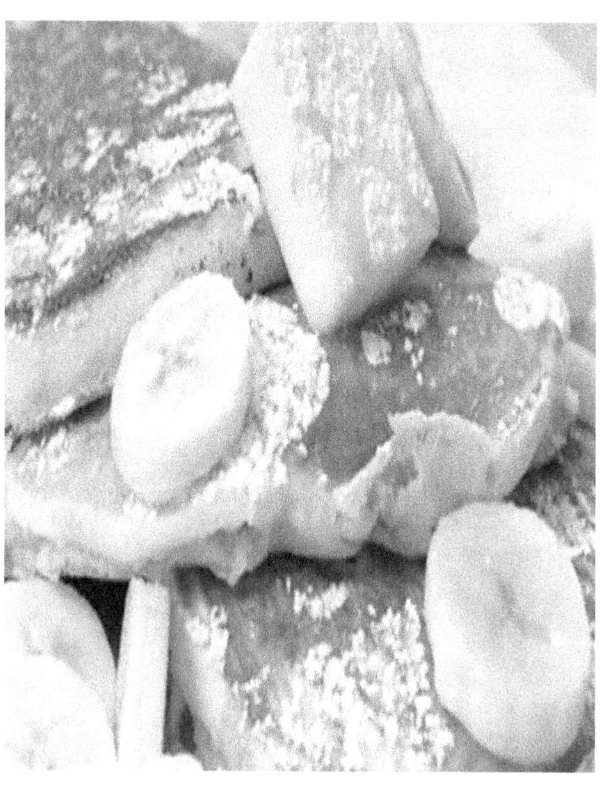

Preparations:

- In a mixing basin, use a fork to mash the ripe banana until smooth.
- Whisk the eggs into the mashed banana until well incorporated.
- If using, add the baking powder and vanilla extract.
- Heat a nonstick pan or griddle over medium heat and gently coat with butter or oil.
- Pour tiny ladlefuls of pancake batter onto the skillet, producing pancakes to your preferred size (typically 3-4 inches in diameter).
- Cook the pancakes for 2-3 minutes on one side, until bubbles appear and the edges begin to firm.
- Flip the pancakes gently and cook for another 1-2 minutes on the other side, until golden brown and thoroughly done.
- Remove the pancakes from the skillet and continue with the remaining batter, greasing the pan as required between batches.
- Serve warm banana pancakes with your favourite toppings, such as fresh berries, sliced bananas, maple syrup, honey, or cinnamon

Nutritional value (Approximate per Serving):

Calories: Approximately 80-100 kcal per pancake (varies based on size)

Protein: 4-5 grams

Fat: 4-5 grams

Saturated Fat: 1-2 grams

Carbohydrates: 8-10 grams

Dietary Fiber: 1-2 grams

Sugars: 5-6 grams (naturally occurring sugars from banana)

Sodium: 60-80 mg

Notes

Your

Observation

Raw brownies

Ingredients:

- 2 ½ cups of pitted fresh Medjool dates
- 1 ½ cups of raw walnuts or pistachios
- 5 tablespoons of cacao or cocoa powder
- 1 tablespoon of canned coconut cream
- ¼ cup of goji berries

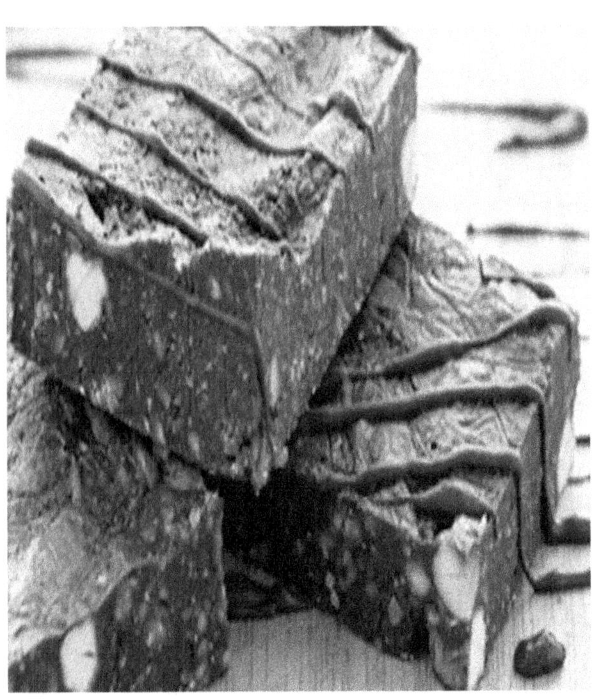

Preparations:

- In a food processor, blend pitted dates, raw walnuts or pistachios, cacao powder, and canned coconut cream.
- Process the ingredients until it has a thick and sticky dough-like consistency. The nuts should be coarsely chopped, and the dates should be well mixed.
- Add the goji berries to the mixture and pulse just to blend. The goji berries will provide a chewy texture and a punch of flavour.
- Line a baking dish or tray with parchment paper to facilitate removal.
- Place the brownie mixture in the prepared baking dish.
- Press the mixture into the dish evenly with your hands or a spatula, smoothing the top.
- Refrigerate the brownie mixture for at least 1-2 hours until set.
- Once cooled and solid, take the brownie slab out of the fridge and cut it into squares or bars.

Nutritional value (Approximate per Serving):

Serving Size: 1 brownie (assuming 12 servings)

Calories: Approximately 200-250 kcal

Protein: 4-5 grams

Fat: 10-12 grams

Saturated Fat: 1-2 grams

Carbohydrates: 30-35 grams

Dietary Fiber: 5-6 grams

Sugars: 25-30 grams (naturally occurring sugars from dates)

Sodium: 5-10 mg

Notes

Your

Observation

CHAPTER 7: SIDES AND SALADS

Baked Salmon With Avocado Salad

Ingredients:

For Baked Salmon:

- 4 salmon fillets (about 6 ounces each), skin-on or skinless
- 2 tablespoons of olive oil
- 1 lemon, thinly sliced
- Salt and pepper, to taste
- Fresh herbs (such as dill, parsley, or thyme), chopped for garnish

For Avocado Salad:

- 2 ripe avocados, diced
- 1 cup of cherry tomatoes, halved
- 1/4 red onion, thinly sliced
- 1 cucumber, diced
- 1 lime, juiced
- 2 tablespoons of extra-virgin olive oil
- Salt and pepper, to taste
- Optional: chopped fresh cilantro or parsley for garnish

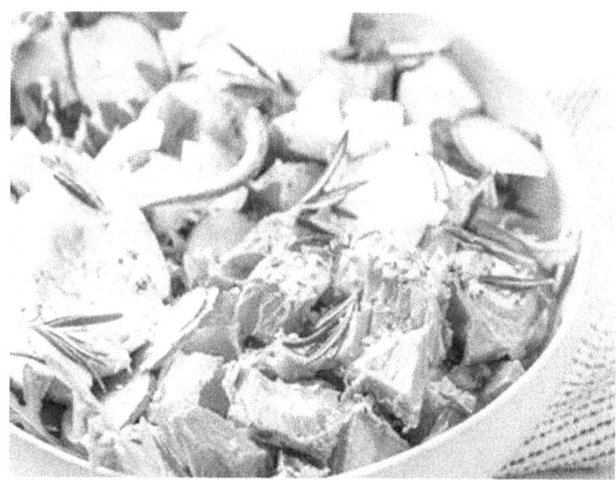

Preparations:

Prepare the baked salmon:

- Preheat the oven to 400 °F (200 °C).
- Place the salmon fillets on a baking pan covered with parchment or aluminium foil.
- Drizzle olive oil over the salmon fillets and season with salt and pepper.
- Place lemon wedges over the salmon fillets.
- Bake the salmon in the preheated oven for 12-15 minutes, or until it is well cooked and readily flaked with a fork.
- Remove from the oven and put aside.

Prepare the avocado salad:

- In a big mixing bowl, add the chopped avocados, cherry tomatoes, red onion, and cucumber.
- Drizzle lime juice and extra virgin olive oil over the salad's components.
- Season with salt and pepper to taste.
- Gently whisk everything together until well incorporated.

Assembly and Service:

- Divide the avocado salad among serving dishes.
- Place one cooked salmon fillet on top of each salad piece.

Garnish with chopped fresh herbs (dill, parsley, or thyme), and optional cilantro or parsley. Serve immediately and enjoy!

Nutritional value(Approximate per Serving):

Calories: Approximately 350-400 kcal (per serving with salmon and salad)

Protein: 30-35 grams

Fat: 20-25 grams

Saturated Fat: 3-4 grams

Carbohydrates: 15-20 grams

Dietary Fiber: 8-10 grams

Sugars: 3-5 grams

Sodium: 300-400 mg

Notes

Your

Observation

Rice and Vegetable Stuffed Capsicums

Ingredients:

- 4 big bell peppers (capsicums), any color
- 1 cup of cooked rice (white or brown)
- 1 cup f mixed vegetables (such as diced carrots, peas, corn, zucchini, or bell pepper)
- 1 small onion, finely chopped
- 2 cloves of minced garlic
- 1 tablespoon of olive oil
- 1 teaspoon of dried herbs (such as thyme, oregano, or basil)
- Salt and pepper, to taste
- 1/2 cup of grated cheese (cheddar, mozzarella, or your choice), optional
- Fresh parsley or cilantro, chopped for
- Garnish

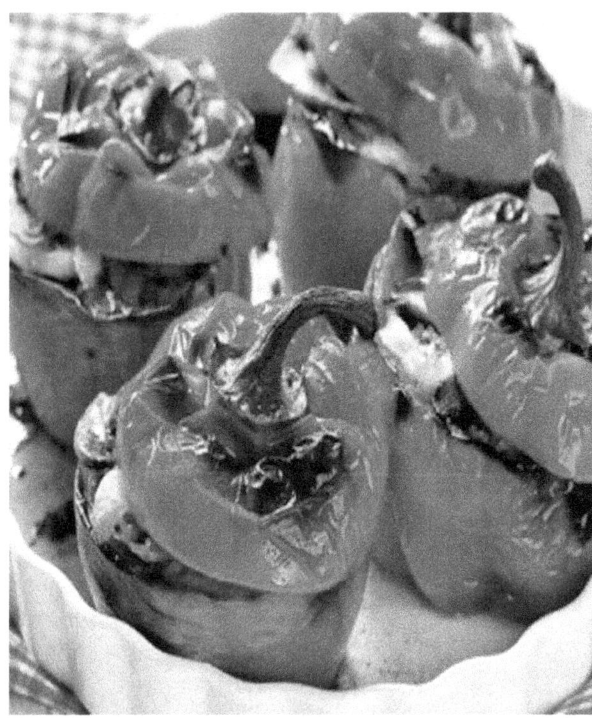

Preaparations:

- To prepare the bell peppers, preheat your oven to 375°F (190°C).
- Cut off the tops of the bell peppers and remove the seeds and membranes from within.
- If necessary, slice a tiny piece off the bottom of each pepper to keep it upright in a baking dish without toppling over.
- Place the hollowed-out bell peppers in a baking dish, upright.
- Prepare the rice and vegetable filling.
- In a skillet or frying pan, heat the olive oil over medium heat.
- Sauté the chopped onion and minced garlic until tender and transparent.
- Add the mixed vegetables to the pan and simmer for a few minutes until they soften.
- Mix in the cooked rice and dry herbs. Season with salt and pepper to taste. Mix everything thoroughly to mix.
- Optional: If using grated cheese, combine half of it with the rice and vegetables.
- To stuff the bell peppers, equally distribute the rice and vegetables mixture and gently push down to pack.
- If preferred, add the leftover grated cheese to the filled peppers.
- To bake stuffed capsicums, cover the baking dish with aluminium foil.
- Place the dish in the preheated oven and cook for 25-30 minutes.
- Remove the foil and bake for another 10-15 minutes, or until the bell peppers are soft and

slightly browned on the edges, and the
mixture is well cooked.

- To serve, remove the stuffed capsicums from the oven and allow them to cool slightly.
- Before serving, garnish with freshly cut parsley or cilantro.
- Serve the rice and vegetable-stuffed capsicums as a tasty and filling vegetarian main course or side dish.

Nutritional value (Approximate per Serving):

Calories: Approximately 200-250 kcal per stuffed capsicum (varies based on size and ingredients)

Protein: 5-8 grams

Fat: 8-10 grams

Saturated Fat: 2-3 grams

Carbohydrates: 30-35 grams

Dietary Fiber: 5-8 grams

Sugars: 5-8 grams

Sodium: 300-400 mg (varies based on seasoning and cheese)

Your

Observation

Tomato Omelette

Ingredients:

- 2 big tomatoes, finely chopped
- 4 eggs
- 1 small onion, finely chopped
- 2-3 green chilies, finely chopped (adjust to taste)
- 1/4 cup of chopped fresh cilantro (coriander)
- 1/2 teaspoon of turmeric powder
- Salt and pepper, to taste
- 2 tablespoons of cooking oil (such as vegetable oil or olive oil)

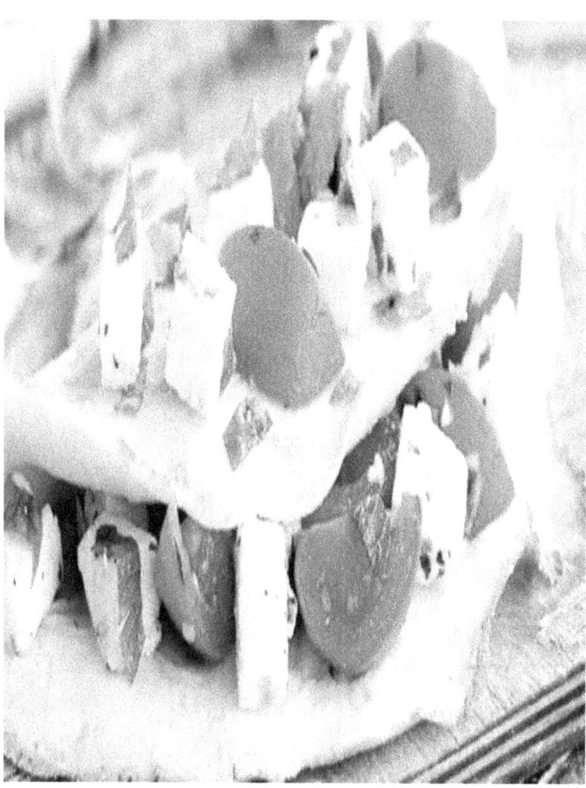

Preparations:

- To make the tomato mixture, combine finely diced tomatoes, onion, green chilies, and cilantro.
- Add the turmeric powder, salt, and pepper to the tomato mixture. Mix well and keep aside.
- Prepare the egg mixture:
- In a separate dish, break the eggs and whisk until thoroughly blended.
- Season the eggs with a touch of salt and pepper.
- *Cooking the tomato omelette:*
- Heat 1 tablespoon oil in a nonstick skillet or frying pan over medium heat.
- Add half of the prepared tomato mixture to the pan and distribute it evenly.
- Cook the tomatoes for around 2-3 minutes, until they soften and release juices.
- Pour half of the whisked eggs equally over the tomato mixture, turning the pan to distribute the eggs.
- Lower the heat to medium-low and cover the skillet. Cook for approximately 3-4 minutes, or until the eggs are set and cooked through.
- Carefully raise the omelette's edges with a spatula to see if the bottom is golden brown and done.
- Once cooked, use a spatula to delicately fold the omelette in half.
- To prepare the second omelette, wipe the skillet with a paper towel and heat the remaining tablespoon of oil over medium heat.

> - Repeat with the remaining tomato mixture and whisked eggs to produce the second omelette.
> - *Serve:*
> - Transfer the cooked tomato omelettes to serving dishes.
> - If desired, garnish with more chopped cilantro.
> - Serve hot alongside toasted bread, chapati, or as a stand-alone meal.

Nutritional value (Approximate per Serving):

Calories: Approximately 200-250 kcal per omelette (varies based on size and ingredients)

Protein: 12-15 grams

Fat: 14-16 grams

Saturated Fat: 3-4 grams

Carbohydrates: 10-12 grams

Dietary Fiber: 3-4 grams

Sugars: 6-8 grams

Sodium: 300-400 mg (varies based on seasoning)

Notes

Your

Observation

Balsamic Roasted Beets

Ingredients:

- 4-5 average-sized beets, peeled and cut into cubes or wedges
- 2 tablespoons of olive oil
- 2 tablespoons of balsamic vinegar
- 1 tablespoon of honey or maple syrup (optional, for added sweetness)
- Salt and pepper, to taste
- Fresh thyme or rosemary sprigs (optional, for garnish)

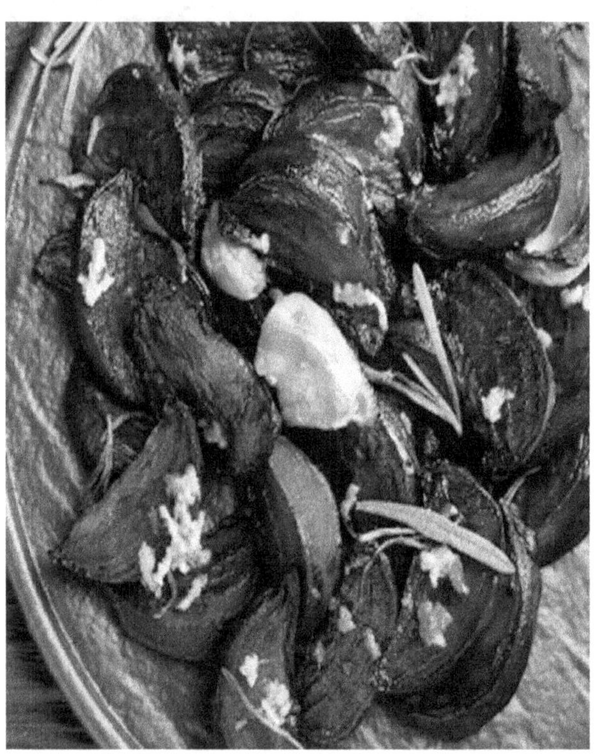

Preparations:

- Preheat the oven to 400°F (200°C) and prepare a baking sheet with parchment paper or aluminium foil.
- Prepare the beets:
- Peel the beets with a vegetable peeler and cut into uniform cubes or wedges.
- Make the balsamic marinade:
- In a mixing bowl, combine olive oil, balsamic vinegar, honey or maple syrup (if using), salt, and pepper.
- Coat the beets.
- Place the diced or wedged beets in the basin with the balsamic marinade.
- Toss the beets until uniformly covered with marinade.
- To roast the beets, spread them in a single layer on a preheated baking sheet.
- Roast the beets for 25-30 minutes, or until soft and caramelised, tossing halfway through to ensure uniform cooking.
- them serve, remove roasted beets from the oven and allow them cool slightly.
- Move the roasted balsamic beets to a serving plate.
- Garnish with thyme or rosemary sprigs, if preferred.

Nutritional value (Approximate per Serving):

Calories: Approximately 100-120 kcal per serving (varies based on serving size and ingredients)

Fat: 7-9 grams

Saturated Fat: 1 gram

Carbohydrates: 10-12 grams

Dietary Fiber: 3-4 grams

Sugars: 7-9 grams

Protein: 1-2 grams

Sodium: 100-150 mg (varies based on seasoning)

Notes

Your

Observation

Coleslaw with Apple Cider Vinaigrette recipe

Ingredients:

- 4 cups of shredded green cabbage
- 1 cup of shredded carrots
- 1/2 cup of mayonnaise (use vegan mayo for a dairy-free option)
- 2 tablespoons of apple cider vinegar
- 1 tablespoon of honey (or maple syrup for vegan option)
- 1 teaspoon of Dijon mustard
- Salt and pepper, to taste
- Chopped fresh parsley or green onions (optional, for garnish)

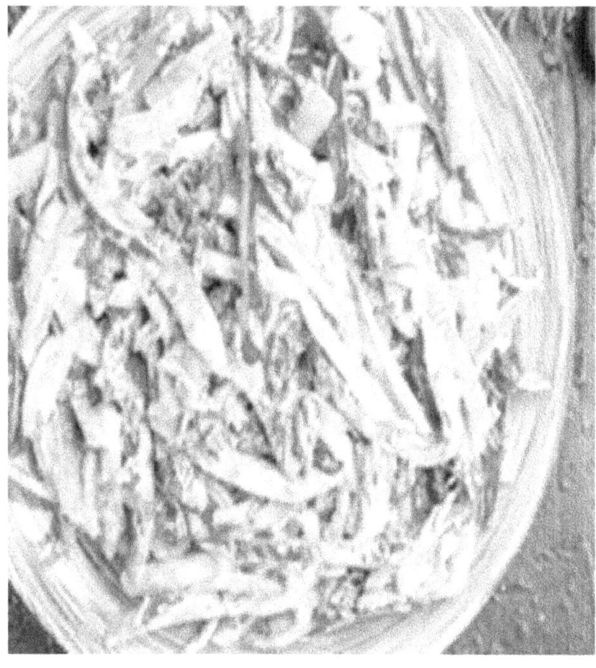

Preparations:

- *Get ready the Vegetables*:
- Using a sharp knife or a food processor, shred the green cabbage and carrots. Put them in a large mixing dish.
- Make the apple cider vinaigrette:
- In a small mixing bowl, combine the mayonnaise, apple cider vinegar, honey (or maple syrup), Dijon mustard, salt, and pepper until smooth and thoroughly blended.
- *Combine the ingredients:*
- Pour the apple cider vinaigrette over the shredded cabbage and carrots in the mixing bowl.
- *Mix well:*
- Toss the coleslaw using salad tongs or a big spoon until the dressing is uniformly distributed among the vegetables.
- *Chill (optional):*
- Cover the coleslaw and chill for at least 30 minutes before serving to enable the flavours to combine.
- To serve and garnish, transfer coleslaw to a serving dish.
- For extra freshness and colour, garnish with chopped fresh parsley or green onions.

Variations:

For added sweetness and texture, add sliced apples or raisins.

Add chopped nuts, such walnuts or almonds, for extra crunch and flavour.

For a more colourful coleslaw, substitute some of the cabbage with shredded red cabbage.

Nutritional value (Per Serving):

Calories: Approximately 150-200 kcal

Fat: 12-15 grams

Saturated Fat: 2-3 grams

Carbohydrates: 10-15 grams

Sugar: 6-8 grams

Protein: 1-2 grams

Fiber: 2-3 grams

Notes

Your

Observation

EAT HEALTHY AND STAY HOPEFUL

CHAPTER 7: DESSERTS

Dairy-Free Cranberry Chocolate Bark

Ingredients:

- 12 ounces of dairy-free dark chocolate (chips or chopped)
- 1/2 cup of dried cranberries
- 1/4 cup of chopped almonds or walnuts
- Optional: flaky sea salt, for sprinkling

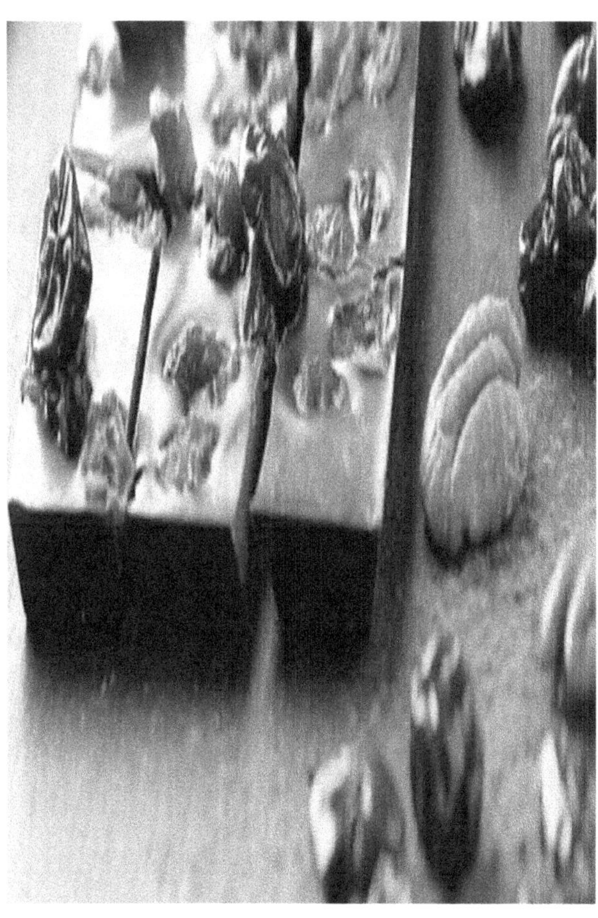

Preparations:

- *Prepare a baking sheet:*
- Line a baking sheet with parchment paper or a silicone baking mat. Set aside.
- To melt the dairy-free dark chocolate, place it in a heatproof dish over simmering water (double boiler method). Stir periodically until smooth and melted.
- Alternatively, microwave the chocolate in 30-second intervals, stirring thoroughly between each, until smooth.
- *Combine Ingredients:*
- Once the chocolate has melted, take the bowl from the heat.
- Quickly whisk in the dried cranberries and chopped almonds or walnuts, keeping a little quantity for topping if preferred.
- To spread the mixture, pour the melted chocolate onto the prepared baking sheet.
- Spread the chocolate evenly, approximately 1/4 inch thick, with a spatula or the back of a spoon.
- Toppings: Sprinkle dried cranberries and chopped nuts on top of the chocolate bark.
- Optional: Sprinkle flaky sea salt over the chocolate bark to create a sweet and salty flavour contrast.

- Chill the baking sheet in the refrigerator for 1 hour to allow the chocolate to set and harden.
- To break into pieces, take the chocolate bark from the refrigerator once it has fully hardened. With a sharp knife, cut or break the bark into pieces of the appropriate size and shape.

- *Serve and enjoy:*
- Serve the dairy-free cranberry chocolate bark as a tasty treat or wrap it in airtight containers for gifts.
- Keep any leftovers in the refrigerator in an airtight container for up to two weeks.

Nutritional value(Approximate per Serving):

Calories: Approximately 150-200 kcal per serving (varies based on serving size)

Fat: 10-12 grams

Saturated Fat: 6-8 grams

Carbohydrates: 15-20 grams

Dietary Fiber: 3-5 grams

Sugars: 10-12 grams

Protein: 2-4 grams

Sodium: 0-50 mg (varies based on chocolate used)

Notes

Your

Observation

Date And Tahini Fudge

Ingredients:

- 1 cup of Medjool dates, pitted (about 10-12 dates)
- 1/2 cup of tahini (sesame seed paste)
- 2 tablespoons of coconut oil, melted
- 1/2 teaspoon of vanilla extract
- Pinch of salt
- Optional toppings: chopped nuts, sesame seeds, or shredded coconut

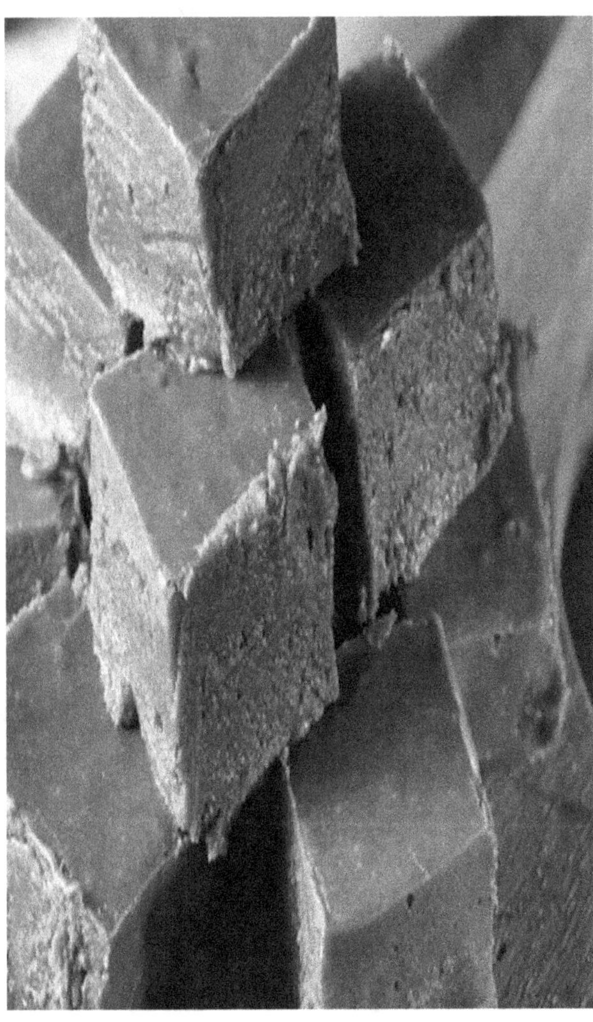

Preparations:

- Prepare the Dates:
- If not already pitted, remove the pits and slice into smaller pieces.
- Blend the ingredients:
- In a food processor or high-speed blender, mix pitted dates, tahini, melted coconut oil, vanilla extract, and a sprinkle of salt.
- Blend until the mixture is smooth and thoroughly incorporated. To achieve equal mixing, you may need to stop the processor or blender and scrape down the sides many times.
- Shape the fudge:
- Line a small baking dish or container with parchment paper, providing enough overhang for easy removal of the fudge.
- Transfer the combined mixture to the prepared dish and use a spatula to distribute it evenly.
- Add optional toppings:
- If preferred, add chopped nuts, sesame seeds, or shredded coconut on top of the fudge and gently press down with your fingertips or the back of a spoon.
- Refrigerate the dish for at least 1-2 hours to allow the fudge to harden up.
- To serve, take the fudge from the refrigerator when it has firmed up.
- Using a sharp knife, cut the fudge into tiny squares or bars.
- Store the date and tahini fudge in an airtight jar in the refrigerator for up to a week.
- Enjoy the fudge as a tasty and healthful snack or dessert

Nutritional value (Approximate per Serving):

Calories: Approximately 100-120 kcal per serving (varies based on serving size)

Fat: 7-9 grams

Saturated Fat: 3-4 grams

Carbohydrates: 8-10 grams

Dietary Fiber: 1-2 grams

Sugars: 6-8 grams

Protein: 2-3 grams

Sodium: 20-30 mg (varies based on ingredients)

Notes

Your

Observation

Natural Vegan Chocolate Bark

Ingredients:

- 10 ounces (about 280 grams) dairy-free dark chocolate (70% cocoa or higher), chopped
- 1/2 cup of chopped nuts (such as almonds, walnuts, pecans)
- 1/4 cup of dried cranberries or other dried fruits (such as cherries, apricots)
- 2 tablespoons of unsweetened shredded coconut
- 1/4 teaspoon of flaky sea salt (optional, for sprinkling)

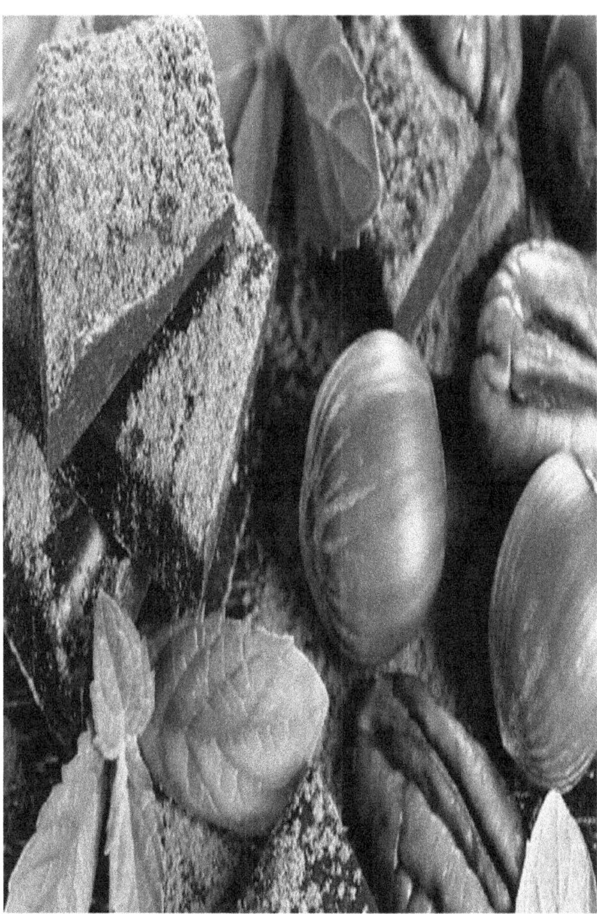

Preparations:

- *Get ready a Baking Sheet:*
- Line a baking sheet with parchment paper or a silicone baking mat. Put aside.
- To melt the dairy-free dark chocolate, place it in a heatproof dish over simmering water (double boiler method). Stir periodically until smooth and melted.
- Alternatively, microwave the chocolate in 30-second intervals, stirring thoroughly between each, until smooth.
- To spread the melted chocolate, pour it over the prepared baking sheet.
- Spread the chocolate evenly, approximately 1/4 inch thick, with a spatula or the back of a spoon.
- *Add toppings:*
- Sprinkle the chopped nuts, dried cranberries (or other dried fruits), and unsweetened shredded coconut over the melted chocolate in an equal layer.
- Gently push the toppings into the chocolate using your fingertips.
- Optional: Add flaky sea salt.
- If desired, sprinkle flaky sea salt over the chocolate bark to create a sweet and salty flavour contrast.
- To chill and set the chocolate, place the baking sheet in the refrigerator for approximately an hour until hard.
- To break into pieces, take the chocolate bark from the refrigerator once it has fully hardened.

- Use a sharp knife or just break the bark into pieces of the desired size and shape.
- *Serve and enjoy:*
- Serve the vegan chocolate bark as a tasty treat or wrap it in airtight containers for giving.
- Keep any leftovers in the refrigerator in an airtight container for up to two weeks.

Nutritional value (Approximate per Serving):

Calories: Approximately 150-200 kcal per serving (varies based on serving size)

Fat: 10-12 grams

Saturated Fat: 6-8 grams

Carbohydrates: 15-20 grams

Dietary Fiber: 3-5 grams

Sugars: 10-12 grams

Protein: 2-4 grams

Sodium: 0-50 mg (varies based on chocolate used)

Notes

Your

Observation

Walnut And Apricot Balls

Ingredients:

- 1 cup of walnuts
- 1 cup of dried apricots (unsweetened), roughly chopped
- 1/2 cup of shredded coconut (unsweetened), plus extra for rolling
- 1 tablespoon of coconut oil, melted
- 1 tablespoon of maple syrup or agave syrup (optional, for added sweetness)
- 1/2 teaspoon of vanilla extract
- Pinch of salt

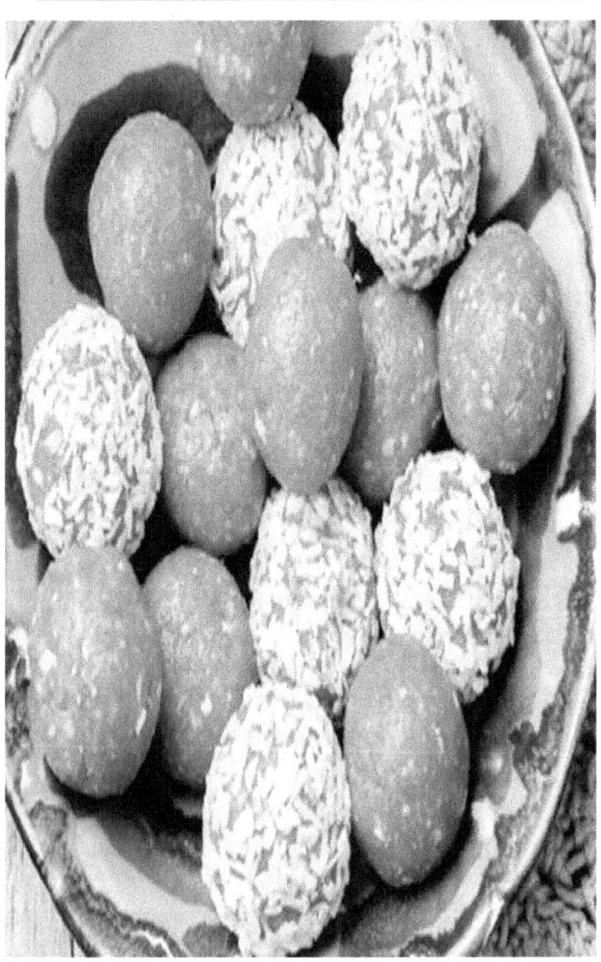

Preparations:

- Prepare the Ingredients:
- If the walnuts are not chopped already, put them in a food processor and pulse until smoothly chopped.
- If the dried apricots haven't previously been sliced, roughly chop them.
- Blend the ingredients:
- In a food processor, mix the chopped walnuts, dried apricots, shredded coconut, melted coconut oil, maple syrup (if using), vanilla essence, and salt.
- Process the ingredients until it has a sticky dough consistency. When you press the mixture between your fingertips, it should stay together.
- To form the balls, scoop out tablespoon-sized quantities of the mixture and roll them into balls with your palms.
- If the mixture is too sticky to handle, gently coat your hands with coconut oil or water.
- To coat each ball equally, roll it in extra shredded coconut.
- Place the coated walnut and apricot balls on a plate or baking sheet covered with parchment paper.
- Refrigerate the walnut and apricot balls for 30 minutes to harden them up.
- Serve cold walnut and apricot balls as a healthful snack or dessert.
- Refrigerate any leftovers in an airtight container for up to a week..

Nutritional value (Approximate per Serving - Makes about 12 balls):

Calories: Approximately 100-120 kcal per ball (varies based on size)

Fat: 7-9 grams

Saturated Fat: 2-3 grams

Carbohydrates: 8-10 grams

Dietary Fiber: 2-3 grams

Sugars: 5-6 grams

Protein: 2-3 grams

Sodium: 5-10 mg

Notes

Your

Observation

JUICING AND SMOOTHIES FOR MASLD

CHAPTER 8: JUICING AND SMOOTHIES

Spring Strawberry Smoothie

Ingredients:

- 1 cup of fresh strawberries, hulled and halved
- 1 ripe banana, peeled and sliced
- 1/2 cup of plain Greek yogurt (or dairy-free yogurt for vegan option)
- 1/2 cup of almond milk (or any preferred milk)
- 1 tablespoon of honey or maple syrup (optional, adjust to taste)
- 1 tablespoon of chia seeds (optional)
- Ice cubes (optional, for a colder smoothie)

Preparations:

- Combine the fresh strawberries, sliced banana, Greek yoghurt, almond milk, and honey or maple syrup (if using) in a blender.
- Add chia seeds for extra nutrition and thickness.
- If you want a cooler smoothie, add a handful of ice cubes to the blender.
- Blend all of the ingredients until smooth and creamy, scraping the sides of the blender as required.
- Taste the smoothie and adjust the sweetness as needed by adding additional honey or maple syrup.
- Pour the spring strawberry smoothie into cups and serve immediately.
- *Optional additions:*
- Add a handful of raw spinach or kale for added nutrition (the smoothie's colour may vary).
- Include a scoop of protein powder for an extra protein boost.
- Garnish with fresh strawberries or mint leaves.

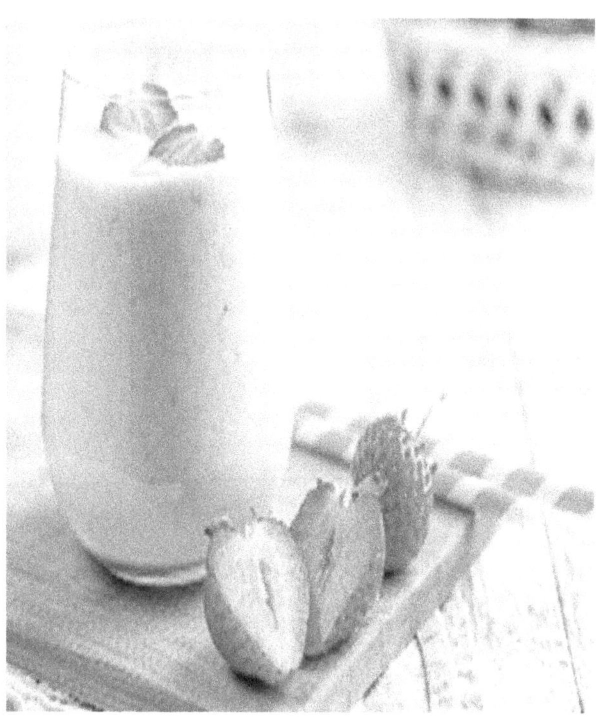

Nutritional Information (Approximate per Serving):

Calories: Approximately 200-250 kcal

Protein: 8-10 grams

Fat: 4-6 grams

Saturated Fat: 1-2 grams

Carbohydrates: 35-40 grams

Dietary Fibre: 5-7 grams

Sugars: 20-25 grams

Calcium: 200-250 mg

Vitamin C: 60-80 mg

Cacao And Almond Smoothie Bowl

Ingredients:

- 1 big ripe banana, frozen
- 1 tablespoon of almond butter
- 1 tablespoon of raw cacao powder
- 1/2 cup of unsweetened almond milk (or any plant-based milk of preference)
- Toppings (optional): sliced almonds, cacao nibs, fresh berries, shredded coconut, granola, chia seeds

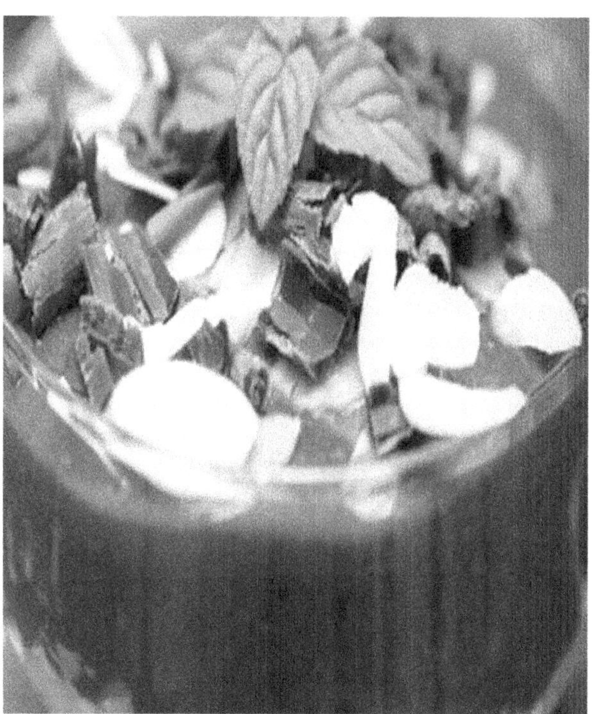

Preparations:

- *Get ready the Smoothie Base:*
- Blend together the frozen banana, almond butter, raw cacao powder, and unsweetened almond milk.
- Blend until smooth.
- Blend the ingredients at high speed until smooth and creamy. If necessary, add additional almond milk gradually to get the required consistency.
- *Pour into a bowl:*
- Pour the cacao-almond smoothie into a bowl.
- *Add toppings:*
- Top the smoothie bowl with sliced almonds, cacao nibs, fresh berries (strawberries or blueberries), shredded coconut, granola, or chia seeds.
- *Serve and enjoy:*
- Serve the cacao and almond smoothie bowl immediately and eat with a spoon

Nutritional value (Approximate per Serving):

Calories: Approximately 300-350 kcal per serving (varies based on ingredients and toppings)

Fat: 15-20 grams

Saturated Fat: 2-3 grams

Carbohydrates: 35-40 grams

Dietary Fiber: 8-10 grams

Sugars: 15-20 grams (naturally occurring from banana)

Protein: 8-10 grams

Sodium: 100-150 mg (varies based on ingredients)

Ginger, Lemon, and Manuka Honey Drink

Ingredients:

- 1-inch piece of fresh ginger, peeled and thinly sliced
- 1 lemon, juiced
- 1 tablespoon of Manuka honey (or raw honey)
- 2 cups of hot water

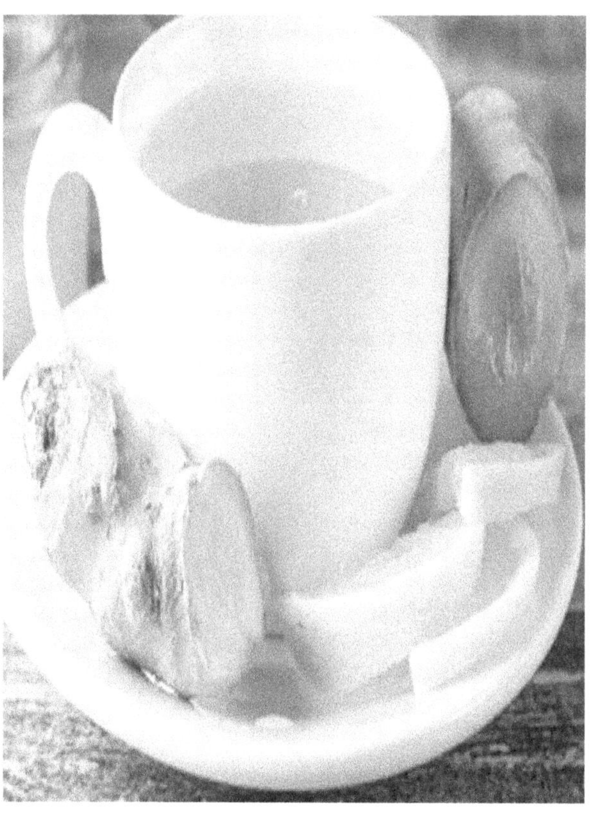

Preparations:

- *Get ready the Ginger:*
- Peel and finely slice 1 inch of fresh ginger.
- Boil 2 cups of water in a kettle or on the hob.
- *Combine Ingredients:*
- Put the sliced ginger in a heatproof mug or cup.
- Squeeze the juice from one lemon into the cup.
- Add 1 tablespoon Manuka honey to the cup.
- *Pour hot water:*
- Carefully pour the boiling water over the ginger, lemon juice, and honey in the cup.
- Steep for 5-10 minutes to infuse the flavours of ginger, lemon, and honey in the water.
- *Stir, and enjoy:*
- Stir the drink until the honey is fully dissolved.
- Sip carefully and relish the calming warmth and flavours of ginger, lemon, and Manuka honey

Benefits:
Ginger is known for its anti-inflammatory effects and ability to calm the digestive tract.
Lemon is high in vitamin C and antioxidants, which can improve immunological health and general well-being.
Manuka honey has natural antibacterial qualities and soothes sore throats and coughs.

Nutritional value:

Calories: Approximately 30-40 kcal per serving (varies based on honey amount)

Carbohydrates: Approximately 9-10 grams (from honey)

Vitamin C: Provides a significant amount of vitamin C from lemon juice

Gingerol (active compound in ginger): Provides anti-inflammatory and antioxidant benefits

Green Detox Smoothie Recipe

Ingredients:

- 3 handfuls of young spinach
- 1 handful of beet leaves (or collard greens), stems removed
- 1 Lebanese cucumber, cut
- 1/2 banana, sliced
- 1 cup of coconut milk (unsweetened)
- 1 tablespoon of chia seeds

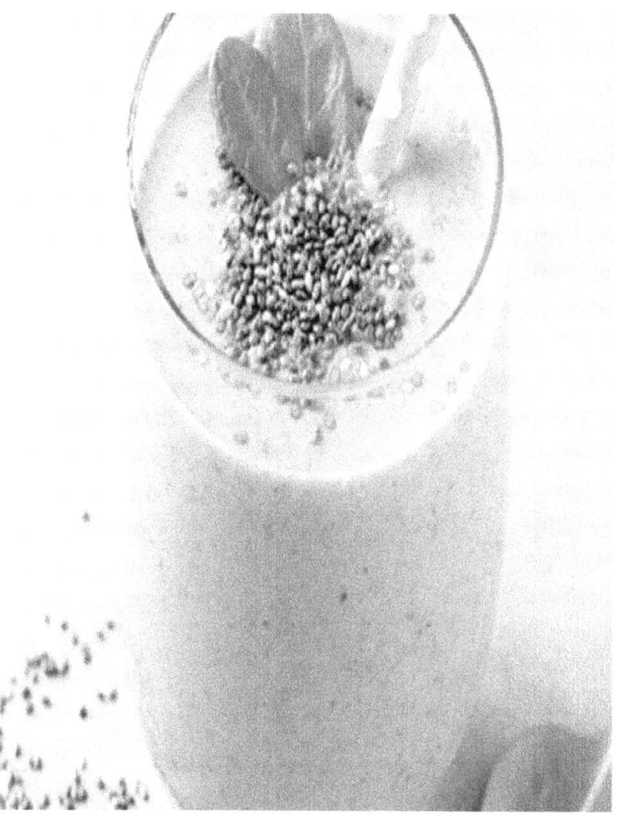

Preparations:

- *Get ready the Ingredients:*
- Rinse the young spinach, beetroot leaves (or collard greens) and Lebanese cucumber completely.
- Cut the cucumber into tiny pieces, then slice the banana.
- *Blend the smoothie:*
- In a blender, add baby spinach, beetroot leaves (or collard greens), cucumber, sliced banana, coconut milk and chia seeds.
- Blend at high speed until all ingredients are fully incorporated and the smoothie has a creamy smoothness.
- *Adjust the consistency (optional):*
- If the smoothie is too thick, add additional coconut milk or water until you get the ideal consistency. If it seems too thin, add additional spinach or banana.
- *Serve and enjoy:*
- Pour the green detox smoothie into the cups.
- Optional garnishes include chia seeds or a sliver of cucumber on the rim

Nutritional Value (Approximate per Serving):

Calories: Approximately 250-300 kcal per serving (varies based on specific ingredients and quantities)

Fat: 15-20 grams

Saturated Fat: 10-12 grams (mainly from coconut milk)

Carbohydrates: 25-30 grams

Dietary Fiber: 8-10 grams

Sugars: 10-12 grams (naturally occurring from fruits and vegetables)

Protein: 5-8 grams

Vitamin A: from spinach and beet leaves

Vitamin C: from spinach, cucumber, and banana

Calcium and Iron: from spinach and chia seeds

Turmeric Almond Milk

Ingredients:

- 1/2 cup of almonds, soaked in water in the fridge overnight
- 2 cups of water
- 1/2 inch of slice fresh turmeric (or 1 teaspoon ground turmeric)
- Pinch of ground cloves
- Liquid stevia, to taste (a few drops)

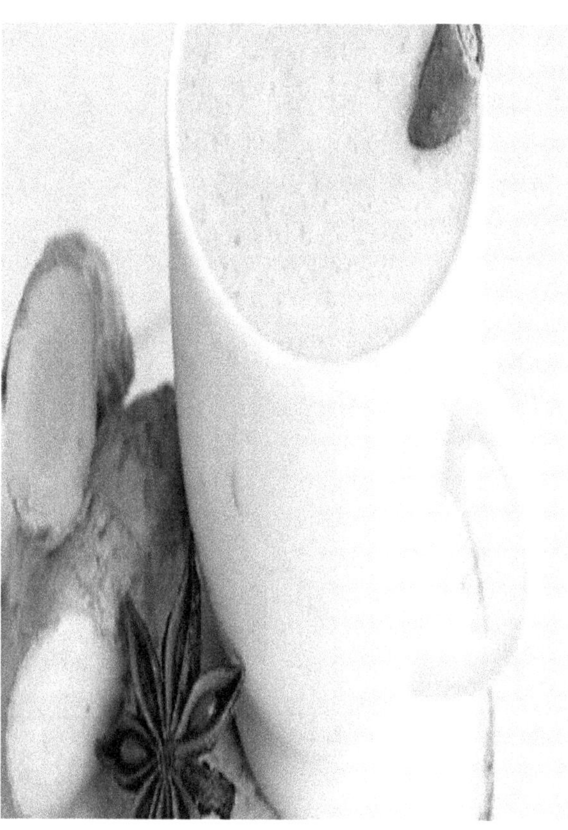

Preparations:

- *Soak the Almonds:*
- To soak almonds, place them in a dish and cover with water. Allow them to soak in the refrigerator overnight, or for at least 8 hours. This softens the almonds for easy mixing.
- *Prepare Turmeric Almond Milk:*
- Drain and rinse the soaked almonds completely.
- In a blender, mix the soaked almonds with 2 cups of water, fresh turmeric (or crushed turmeric), and a pinch of ground cloves.
- *Blend until smooth:*
- Blend on high speed for 1-2 minutes, or until the almonds are well incorporated and the mixture seems creamy.
- Optional: To remove almond pulp, drain the blended almond mixture using a nut milk bag, cheesecloth, or fine mesh sieve. This step is optional if you want a smoother texture.
- To warm and sweeten, pour strained almond milk into a small pot.
- Heat the almond milk on medium-low heat until it is warm but not boiling.
- Add a few drops of liquid stevia and adjust the sweetness to taste.
- Pour heated turmeric almond milk into glasses or cups.
- Enjoy this calming beverage as a soothing treat.

Nutritional Value (Approximate per Serving):

Calories: Approximately 150-200 kcal per serving (varies based on specific ingredients and quantities)

Fat: 12-15 grams

Saturated Fat: 1-2 grams

Carbohydrates: 6-8 grams

Dietary Fiber: 2-3 grams

Sugars: 1-2 grams (naturally occurring from almonds)

Protein: 5-7 grams

Vitamin E: from almonds

Iron and Calcium: from almonds

Creamy Peach Smoothie

- 1 cup of ripe peach slices (fresh or frozen)
- 1/2 cup of plain Greek yogurt (or dairy-free yogurt for vegan option)
- 1/2 cup of almond milk (or any milk of preference)
- 1 tablespoon of honey (or maple syrup for vegan option)
- 1/2 teaspoon of vanilla extract
- Ice cubes (if using fresh peach slices)
- Optional: a sprinkle of ground cinnamon or nutmeg for extra flavor

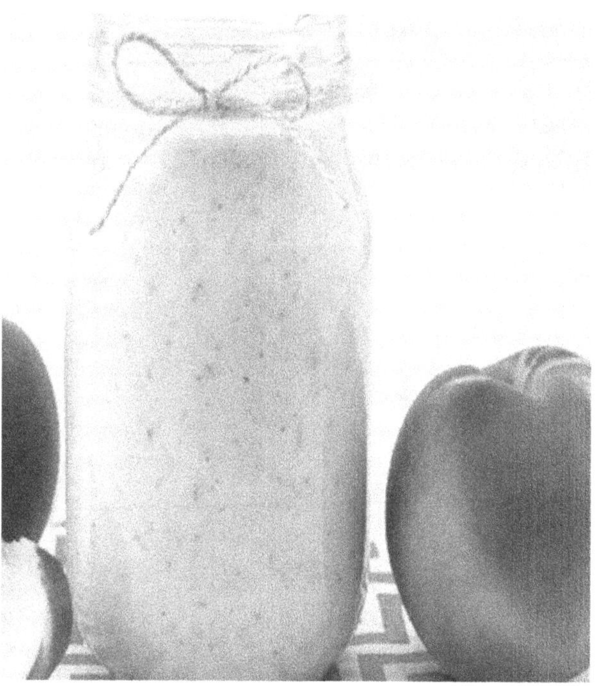

Preparations:

- *Get ready the Peaches:*
- For fresh peaches, wash, pit, and slice into pieces. If you're using frozen peaches, measure out 1 cup of frozen slices.
- *Blend the ingredients:*
- Blend together the peach pieces, Greek yoghurt, almond milk, honey (or maple syrup), and vanilla essence.
- If you use fresh peaches and want a cooler smoothie, add a few ice cubes to the blender.
- *Blend until smooth:*
- Blend the ingredients at high speed until smooth and creamy. If the consistency is too thick, gently add additional almond milk until you get the correct thickness.
- *Taste and adjust:*
- Taste the peach smoothie and adjust the sweetness as required by adding additional honey or maple syrup.
- *Serve and enjoy:*
- Pour the creamy peach smoothie into the cups.
- For added flavour, sprinkle with ground cinnamon or nutmeg

Nutritional value (Approximate per Serving):

Calories: Approximately 150-200 kcal per serving (varies based on specific ingredients and quantities)

Fat: 4-6 grams

Saturated Fat: 1-2 grams

Carbohydrates: 25-30 grams

Dietary Fiber: 3-4 grams

Sugars: 20-25 grams (naturally occurring from peaches and yogurt)

Protein: 8-10 grams

Vitamin C: from peaches

Calcium and Probiotics: from Greek yogurt

Alkalizing Green Juice

Ingredients:

- 1 big handful spinach leaves
- 2 red radishes
- 1 lime, peeled
- 1 green apple, cored and sliced
- 1 big handful parsley
- 1 average cucumber, chopped

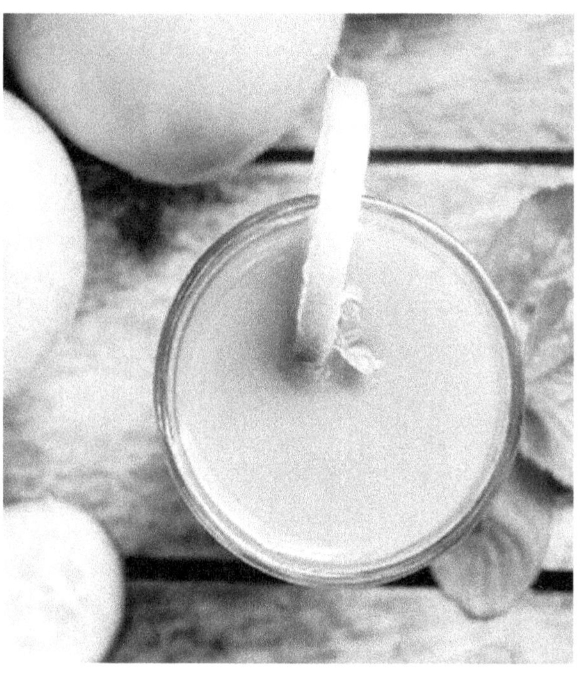

Preparations:

- *Get ready the Ingredients:*
- Wash all fresh fruit thoroughly with running water.
- Core and slice the green apple. Peel a lime.
- Chop the cucumber into tiny pieces.
- *Juicing Process:*
- Begin by juicing the spinach leaves, radishes, lime, green apple, parsley, and cucumber.
- Feed each item into the juicer using the proper settings.
- *Mix well:*
- Once all of the ingredients have been juiced, thoroughly whisk the green juice to integrate the flavours.
- *Serve and enjoy:*
- Pour the alkalizing green juice into the glasses.
- Serve with ice for a cold beverage.

Nutritional Value (Approximate per Serving):

Calories: Approximately 100-120 kcal per serving (varies based on specific ingredients and quantities)

Fat: 0-1 grams

Saturated Fat: 0 grams

Carbohydrates: 25-30 grams

Dietary Fiber: 6-8 grams

Sugars: 15-20 grams (naturally occurring from fruits and vegetables)

Protein: 3-4 grams

Vitamin A: from spinach and parsley

Vitamin C: from lime, radishes, and cucumber

Potassium and Magnesium: from cucumber and parsley

Immune Boosting Raw Juice Recipe

Ingredients:

- 2 stalks celery
- 1/4 red onion
- 2 red radishes
- 2 cabbage leaves
- 1 big carrot
- 2-inch slice of pineapple

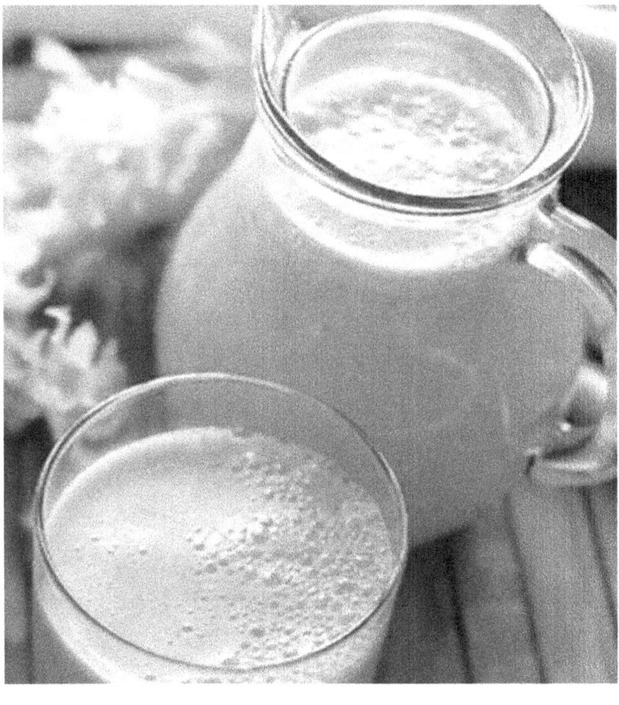

Preparations:

- *Prepare the Ingredients:*
- Wash all fresh fruit thoroughly with running water.
- Trim the celery stalks' ends and chop them into little pieces.
- Peel and cut the red onion into bits.
- Trim the radishes' ends and slice them.
- Tear the cabbage leaves into tiny pieces.
- Peel and chop the carrot into manageable bits.
- Cut the pineapple slice into bits and remove the outer shell.
- *Juicing Process:*
- Begin with juicing the celery, then add the red onion, radishes, cabbage leaves, carrot, and pineapple.
- Feed each item into the juicer using the proper settings.
- *Mix well:*
- To mix the flavours, thoroughly stir the immune-boosting raw juice.
- *Serve and enjoy:*
- Pour raw juice into glasses.
- Serve over ice for a refreshing drink.

Nutritional Value (Approximate per Serving):

Calories: Approximately 80-100 kcal per serving (depends on specific ingredients and quantities)

Fat: 0-1 grams

Saturated Fat: 0 grams

Carbohydrates: 20-25 grams

Dietary Fiber: 5-8 grams

Sugars: 12-15 grams (naturally occurring from fruits and vegetables)

Protein: 2-3 grams

Vitamin C: From pineapple, radishes, and cabbage

Vitamin A: From carrot and cabbage

Potassium: From celery and pineapple

Chocolate And Hazelnut Protein Smoothie

Ingredients:

- 1 frozen banana, chopped (cut it before freezing)
- 1 tablespoon of hazelnut butter
- 1 tablespoon of cocoa or cacao powder
- 2 tablespoons of whey protein powder (or plant-based protein powder for vegan option)
- 1 tablespoon of chia seeds
- 1 glass of water or milk of your choice (almond milk, oat milk, or dairy milk)

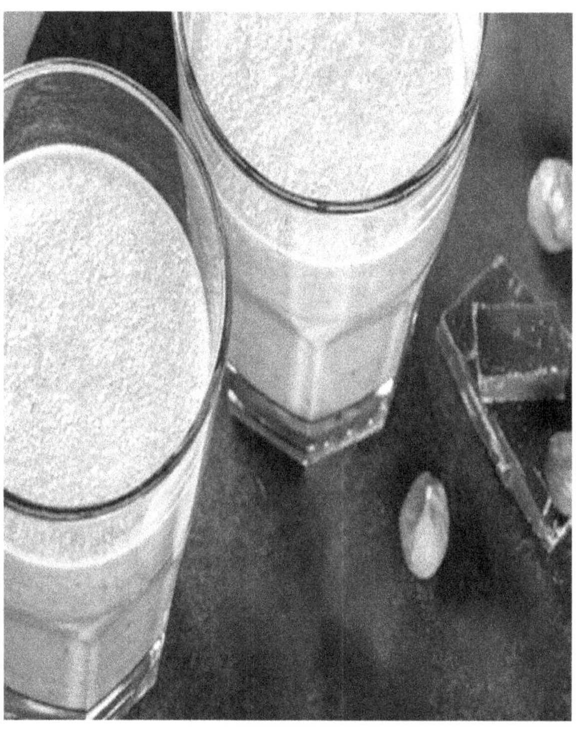

Preparations:

- *Get ready the Ingredients:*
- Cut and freeze the banana. This gives your smoothie a creamy texture without the need for ice.
- Measure the hazelnut butter, cocoa or cacao powder, whey protein powder, and chia seeds.
- *Blend the smoothie:*
- In a blender, add the frozen chopped banana, hazelnut butter, chocolate or cacao powder, whey protein powder, chia seeds, and your preferred water or milk.
- *Blend until smooth:*
- Blend all of the ingredients at high speed until smooth and creamy. Add extra water or milk as needed to get the desired consistency.
- To alter the smoothie's sweetness or thickness, add additional hazelnut butter, cocoa powder, or sweetener as needed.
- *Serve and enjoy:*
- Pour the chocolate-hazelnut protein smoothie into a glass.
- Optionally, put chocolate powder or broken hazelnuts on top.

Nutritional Value (Approximate per Serving):

Calories: Approximately 300-350 kcal per serving (depends on specific ingredients and quantities)

Fat: 12-15 grams

Saturated Fat: 2-3 grams

Carbohydrates: 35-40 grams

Dietary Fiber: 8-10 grams

Sugars: 15-20 grams (naturally occurring from banana and cocoa)

Protein: 15-20 grams

Calcium and Iron: From whey protein powder and chia seeds

Nectarine Smoothie

Ingredients:

- 1 big nectarine, pitted and sliced
- 2 tablespoons of canned coconut cream
- 1 tablespoon of ground flaxseeds
- 2 tablespoons of whey protein powder (or plant-based protein powder for vegan option)
- 1.5 cups of water (adjust amount based on preferred thickness)

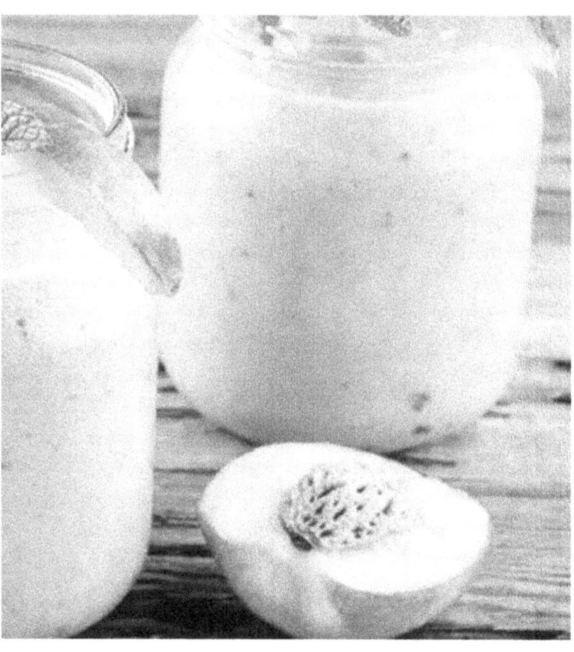

Preparations:

- *Get ready the Ingredients:*
- Wash, pit, and slice the nectarines.
- Measure the canned coconut cream, ground flaxseeds, whey protein powder, and water.
- *Blend the smoothie:*
- In a blender, add sliced nectarine, canned coconut cream, ground flaxseeds, whey protein powder, and water.
- *Blend until smooth:*
- Blend all of the ingredients at high speed until smooth and well incorporated. Add extra water as needed to get the desired consistency.
- *Taste and adjust:*
- Taste the smoothie and adjust the sweetness or thickness as needed by adding more nectarine, coconut cream, or sweetener.
- *Serve and enjoy:*
- Pour the summer nectarine smoothie into individual glasses.
- Optional garnishes include a nectarine slice or a sprinkling of ground flaxseeds.

Nutritional Value (Approximate per Serving):

Calories: Approximately 250-300 kcal per serving (depends on specific ingredients and quantities)

Fat: 12-15 grams

Saturated Fat: 8-10 grams (mainly from coconut cream)

Carbohydrates: 20-25 grams

Dietary Fiber: 4-6 grams

Sugars: 10-15 grams (naturally occurring from nectarine)

Protein: 15-20 grams

Omega-3 Fatty Acids: From ground flaxseeds

Vitamin C and Calcium: From whey protein powder

Cacao And Banana Thick Shake

Ingredients:

- 2 tablespoons of cacao (or cocoa) powder
- 1 chopped frozen banana
- 3 tablespoons of whey protein powder (or plant-based protein powder for vegan option)
- 1 tablespoon of almond butter
- 1 cup of almond milk
- Cacao nibs to sprinkle on top (optional, for garnish)

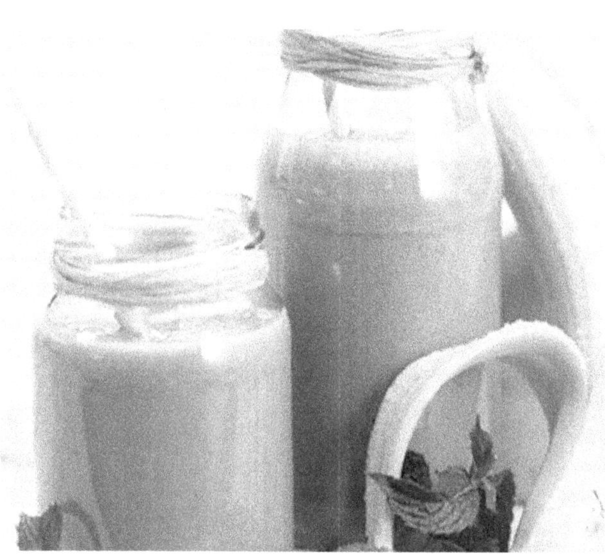

Preparations:

- *Get ready the Ingredients:*
- To achieve a creamier texture, chop a ripe banana into pieces and freeze it beforehand.
- Measure the cacao powder, whey protein powder, almond butter, and almond milk.
- *Blend the thick shake*:
- Blend together the frozen banana chunks, cacao powder, whey protein powder, almond butter, and almond milk.
- *Blend until smooth and creamy:*
- Blend all of the ingredients at high speed until smooth and creamy. Scrape the sides of the blender as needed to ensure that everything is well blended.
- Optional: If the shake is too thick, add additional almond milk and mix again to achieve the ideal consistency.
- *Serve and garnish*:
- Pour the cacao-banana thick shake into a glass.
- Sprinkle cacao nibs on top for extra texture and chocolate flavour.

Nutritional Value (Approximate per Serving):

Calories: Approximately 350-400 kcal per serving (Depends on specific ingredients and quantities)

Fat: 15-20 grams

Saturated Fat: 2-3 grams

Carbohydrates: 30-35 grams

Dietary Fiber: 7-9 grams

Sugars: 15-20 grams (naturally occurring from banana and almond milk)

Protein: 25-30 grams

Calcium and Iron: From almond milk and whey protein powder

Apple And Cinnamon Smoothie

Ingredients:

- 1 big apple, cored and chopped
- 1/2 teaspoon of ground cinnamon
- 1 tablespoon of almond butter (or peanut butter)
- 1 tablespoon of honey (or maple syrup for vegan option)
- 1 cup of almond milk (or any milk of your choice)
- Ice cubes (optional, for a chilled smoothie)

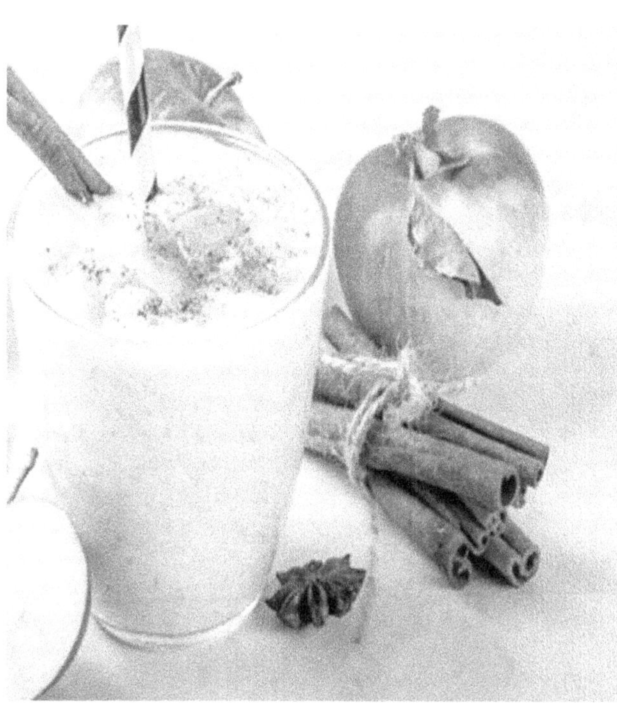

Preparations:

- *Get ready the Ingredients:*
- Wash, core, and cut the apples into bits.
- Measure the ground cinnamon, almond butter, honey (or maple syrup), and almond milk.
- *Blend the smoothie:*
- In a blender, add the diced apples, ground cinnamon, almond butter, honey (or maple syrup), and almond milk.
- If you want a chilly smoothie, add a few ice cubes.
- *Blend until smooth:*
- Blend all of the ingredients at high speed until smooth and creamy. Scrape the sides of the blender as needed to ensure that everything is well blended.
- *Taste and adjust:*
- Taste the smoothie and alter the sweetness or cinnamon flavour to your pleasure. If desired, add extra honey or cinnamon.
- *Serve and enjoy:*
- Pour the apple cinnamon smoothie into glasses.
- Sprinkle a dash of ground cinnamon on top as a garnish.

Nutritional Value (Approximate per Serving):

Calories: Approximately 200-250 kcal per serving (Depends on specific ingredients and quantities)

Fat: 8-10 grams

Saturated Fat: 1-2 grams

Carbohydrates: 30-35 grams

Dietary Fiber: 5-7 grams

Sugars: 20-25 grams (naturally occurring from apple and honey)

Protein: 4-6 grams

Vitamin C: From apple

Calcium and Iron: From almond milk

Creamy Pumpkin Smoothie

Ingredients:

- 1/2 cup of cooked mashed pumpkin (canned pumpkin puree works too)
- 2 tablespoons of whey protein powder (or plant-based protein powder for vegan option)
- 1 tablespoon of chia seeds
- 1 tablespoon of almond butter
- 1/4 teaspoon of pumpkin spice powder (or a combination of cinnamon, nutmeg, and cloves)
- 1.5 cups of water or coconut milk (adjust amount based on preferred thickness)

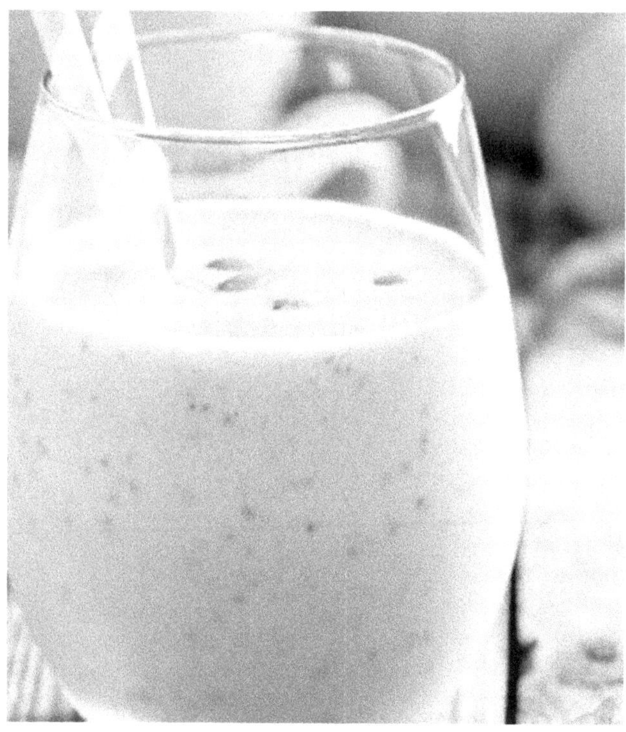

Preparations:

- *Get ready the Ingredients*:
- For fresh pumpkin, simmer and mash until smooth. For added convenience, you may use canned pumpkin puree.
- Measure out the whey protein powder, chia seeds, almond butter, pumpkin spice powder, and water/coconut milk.
- To make the smoothie, mix cooked mashed pumpkin (or canned pumpkin), whey protein powder, chia seeds, almond butter, pumpkin spice powder, and water or coconut milk.
- Start with less liquid to achieve a thicker consistency, then add more as required.
- *Blend until smooth and creamy:*
- Blend all of the ingredients at high speed until smooth and well incorporated. Scrape down the edges of the blender as needed to ensure that everything is mixed evenly.
- Optional: If the smoothie is too thick, add extra water or coconut milk and mix again to achieve the desired consistency.
- *Serve and enjoy:*
- Pour the creamy pumpkin smoothie into individual glasses.
- Sprinkle a pinch of pumpkin spice on top as a garnish

Nutritional Value (Approximate per Serving):

Calories: Approximately 300-350 kcal per serving (Depends on specific ingredients and quantities)

Fat: 15-20 grams

Saturated Fat: 2-3 grams

Carbohydrates: 20-25 grams

Dietary Fiber: 7-9 grams

Sugars: 5-8 grams (naturally occurring from pumpkin and almond butter)

Protein: 20-25 grams

Vitamin A and Vitamin C: From pumpkin

Calcium and Iron: From whey protein powder and chia seeds

Coconut and strawberry smoothie

Ingredients:

- 1 cup of strawberries (fresh or frozen), hulled
- 1/2 cup of coconut milk (canned or from a carton)
- 1/2 cup of plain Greek yogurt (or dairy-free yogurt for vegan option)
- 1 tablespoon of honey (or maple syrup for vegan option)
- Ice cubes (optional, for a chilled smoothie)
- Fresh mint leaves for garnish (optional)

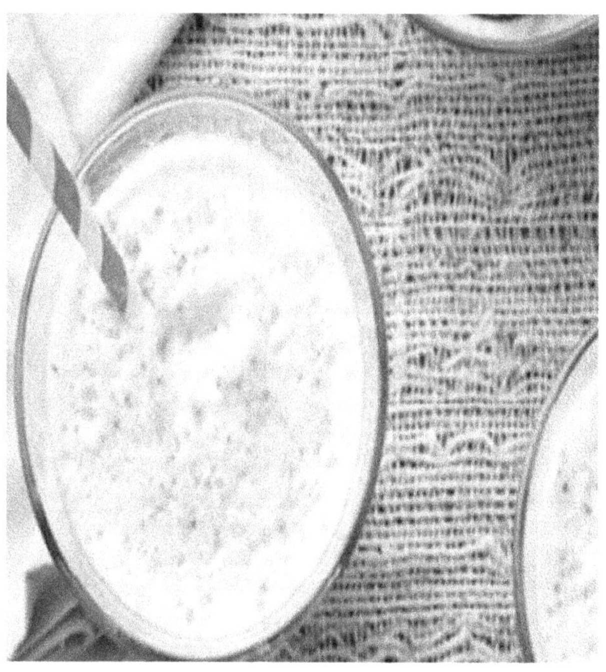

Preparations:

- *Get ready the Ingredients:*
- Wash and hull strawberries, removing the stems.
- Prepare the coconut milk, Greek yoghurt, honey (or maple syrup), and ice cubes (if desired).
- *Blend the smoothie:*
- In a blender, mix strawberries, coconut milk, Greek yoghurt, and honey (or maple syrup).
- If you want your smoothie chilly, add a handful of ice cubes.
- *Blend until smooth:*
- Blend all of the ingredients at high speed until smooth and well incorporated. Scrape down the edges of the blender as needed to ensure that everything is mixed evenly.
- To adjust sweetness, taste the smoothie and add additional honey or maple syrup as needed.
- *Serve and garnish:*
- Pour the coconut-strawberry smoothie into glasses.
- Garnish with fresh mint leaves for a burst of colour and flavour.

Nutritional Value (Approximate per Serving):

Calories: Approximately 150-200 kcal per serving (Depends on specific ingredients and quantities)

Fat: 8-10 grams

Saturated Fat: 6-8 grams (mainly from coconut milk)

Carbohydrates: 15-20 grams

Dietary Fiber: 2-4 grams

Sugars: 10-15 grams (naturally occurring from strawberries and honey)

Protein: 5-8 grams

Vitamin C: From strawberries

Calcium and Probiotics: From Greek yogurt

Anti-Inflammatory Green smoothie

Ingredients:

- 2 handfuls of collard greens or bok choy
- 2 handfuls of parsley
- 1 handful of kale leaves
- 1 small cucumber, chopped
- 1 kiwi fruit, peeled and sliced
- 1 cup of water
- 1 tablespoon of coconut oil

Preparations:

- Get ready the Ingredients:
- Rinse the collard greens (or bok choy), parsley, kale leaves, cucumber, and kiwi fruit well.
- Remove the rough stems from the collard greens and kale leaves.
- To make the smoothie, mix together collard greens (or bok choy), parsley, kale leaves, diced cucumber, sliced kiwi fruit, water, and coconut oil.
- Blend until smooth:
- Blend all of the ingredients at high speed until smooth and well incorporated. Add extra water as needed to get the desired consistency.
- To enhance the smoothie's flavour, add extra fruit (e.g., kiwi) for sweetness or more greens for an antioxidant boost.
- Serve and enjoy:
- Pour the anti-inflammatory green smoothie into the cups.
- Optional garnishes include a piece of kiwi or a sprig of parsley.

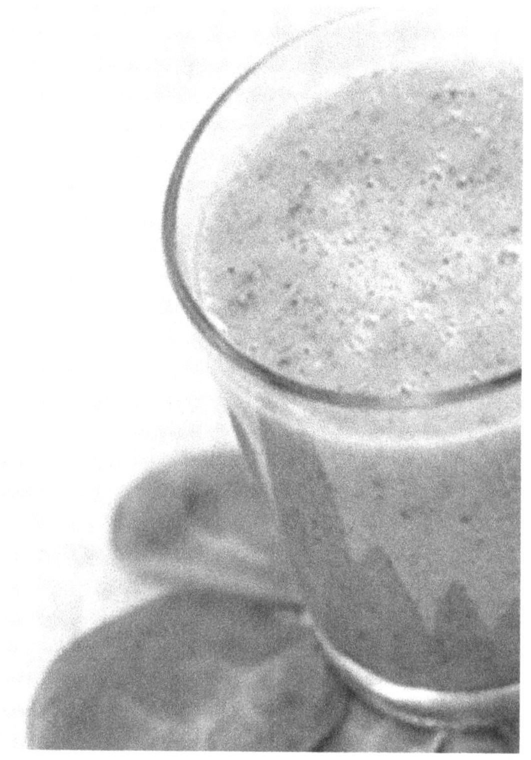

Nutritional Value (Approximate per Serving):

Calories: Approximately 150-200 kcal per serving (Depends on specific ingredients and quantities)

Fat: 10-12 grams

Saturated Fat: 7-9 grams (mainly from coconut oil)

Carbohydrates: 15-20 grams

Dietary Fiber: 5-8 grams

Sugars: 7-10 grams (naturally occurring from fruits and vegetables)

Protein: 5-7 grams

Vitamin C and Vitamin K: From parsley, kale, and kiwi fruit

Omega-3 Fatty Acids: From coconut oil

Notes

Your

Observation

Notes

Your

Observation

CHAPTER 9: 10 DAY MEAL PLANNING

Day 1:

Breakfast: Creamy Pumpkin Smoothie

Lunch: Green Salad with Grilled Chicken

Dinner: Baked Salmon with Avocado Salad

Day 2:

Breakfast: Coconut and Strawberry Smoothie

Lunch: Quinoa Salad with Roasted Vegetables

Dinner: Tomato Omelette with Sautéed Spinach

Day 3:

Breakfast: Cacao and Banana Thick Shake

Lunch: Rice and Vegetable Stuffed Capsicums

Dinner: Shrimp and Broccoli Stir Fry

Day 4:

Breakfast: Anti-Inflammatory Green Smoothie (Collards, Parsley, Kale, Cucumber, Kiwi, Coconut Oil)

Lunch: Lentil Soup with Whole Grain Bread

Dinner: Roasted Broccoli with Pine Nuts and Grilled Chicken

Day 5:

Breakfast: Creamy Peach Smoothie

Lunch: Turkey Lettuce Wraps with Raw Carrot and Almond Salad

Dinner: Baked Lime and Chilli Chicken with Steamed Vegetables

Day 6:

Breakfast: Warm Turmeric Almond Milk

Lunch: Gluten-Free Cinnamon Rice Porridge

Dinner: Low Carb Lamb Stew

Day 7:

Breakfast: Apple and Cinnamon Smoothie

Lunch: Chickpea Salad with Lemon-Tahini Dressing

Dinner: Sugar-Free Beef Ginger Stir Fry

Day 8:

Breakfast: Coconut and Strawberry Smoothie

Lunch: Tomato Omelette with Balsamic Roasted Beets

Dinner: Roast Pumpkin and Cumin Hummus with Raw Carrot and Almond Salad

Day 9:

Breakfast: Green Smoothie to Detox (Spinach, Radish, Apple, Cucumber, Parsley)

Lunch: Chicken Quinoa Bowl with Avocado and Cherry Tomatoes

Dinner: Walnut and Apricot Balls with Side Salad

Day 10:

Breakfast: Anti-Inflammatory Green Smoothie (Collards, Parsley, Kale, Cucumber, Kiwi, Coconut Oil)

Lunch: Greek Salad with Grilled Salmon

Dinner: Grilled Peaches and Feta Salad

CHAPTER 10: CONCLUSION

The MASLD diet cookbook is an invaluable resource for anyone looking to control metabolic dysfunction-associated steatotic liver disease (MASLD) with dietary changes. This cookbook emphasises the significance of eating a liver-friendly diet that includes whole foods, healthy fats, lean proteins, and low-glycemic carbs while limiting processed foods, sweets, and bad fats.

The meals in the MASLD diet cookbook are particularly intended to improve liver function and reduce inflammation, addressing important aspects that contribute to MASLD. This cookbook offers practical and tasty meal alternatives by using nutrient-dense items including leafy greens, cruciferous veggies, lean meats, and anti-inflammatory spices.

Furthermore, the MASLD diet cookbook emphasises the need of personalised nutrition and lifestyle adjustments in treating MASLD. It encourages people to collaborate closely with healthcare providers and nutritionists to customise nutritional plans based on their own requirements and preferences.

Finally, following a MASLD-friendly diet can help with liver function, fat deposition in the liver, and general metabolic health. To effectively control MASLD, dietary adjustments must be supplemented with frequent physical exercise and other lifestyle changes.

In essence, the MASLD diet cookbook is a thorough guide for anyone wishing to improve their diet and nutrition in order to maintain liver function and effectively manage MASLD. Individuals who embrace the concepts and dishes contained in this cookbook can take proactive measures towards improving their health and general well-being.

STAY HEALTHY!

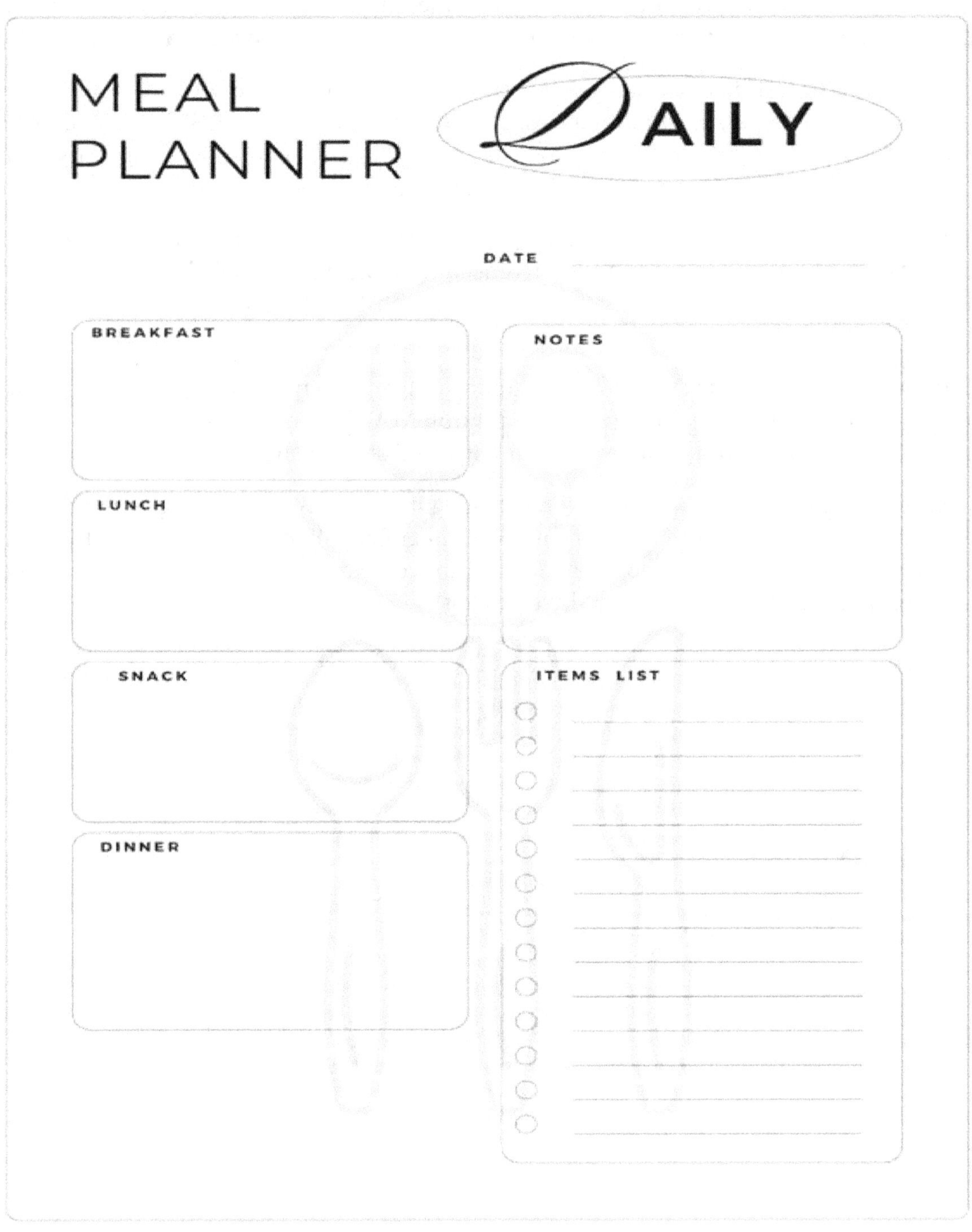
MEAL PLANNER
DAILY
DATE
BREAKFAST
NOTES
LUNCH
SNACK
ITEMS LIST
DINNER

MEAL PLANNER

*D*AILY

DATE

BREAKFAST

NOTES

LUNCH

SNACK

ITEMS LIST

DINNER

MEAL PLANNER

*D*AILY

DATE

BREAKFAST

LUNCH

SNACK

DINNER

NOTES

ITEMS LIST

MEAL PLANNER

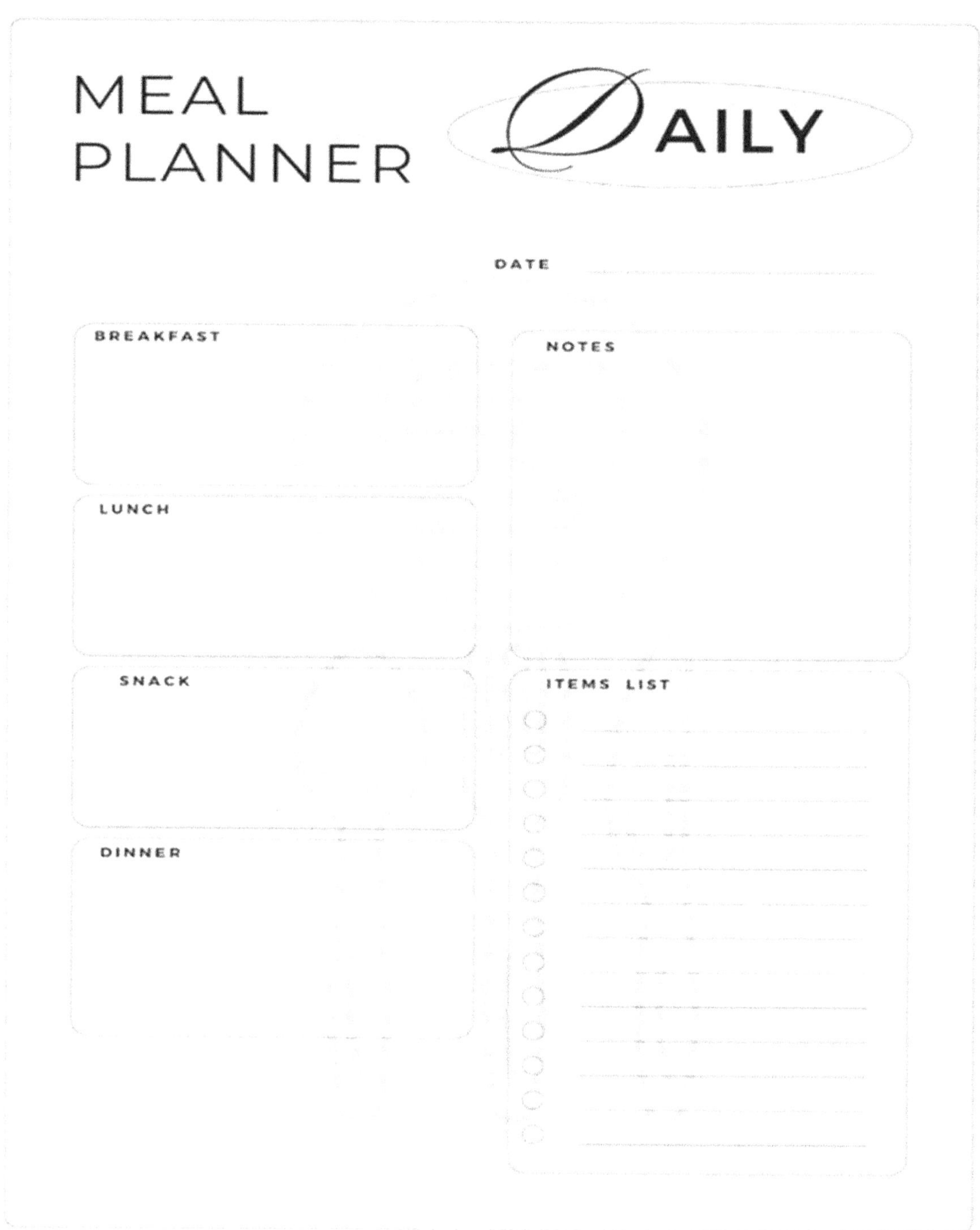

MEAL PLANNER

DAILY

DATE ___________________

BREAKFAST

LUNCH

SNACK

DINNER

NOTES

ITEMS LIST

MEAL PLANNER

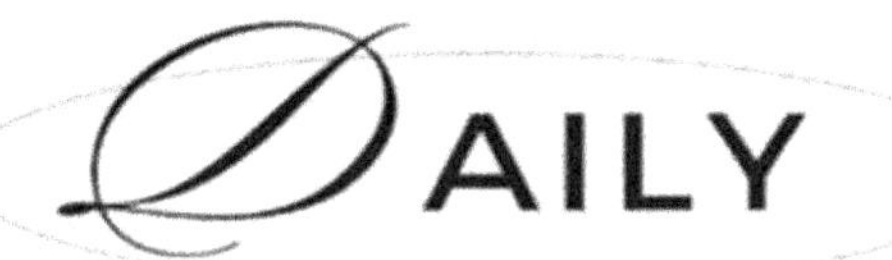

DATE

BREAKFAST

LUNCH

SNACK

DINNER

NOTES

ITEMS LIST

MEAL PLANNER

DAILY

DATE

BREAKFAST

NOTES

LUNCH

SNACK

ITEMS LIST

DINNER

MEAL PLANNER

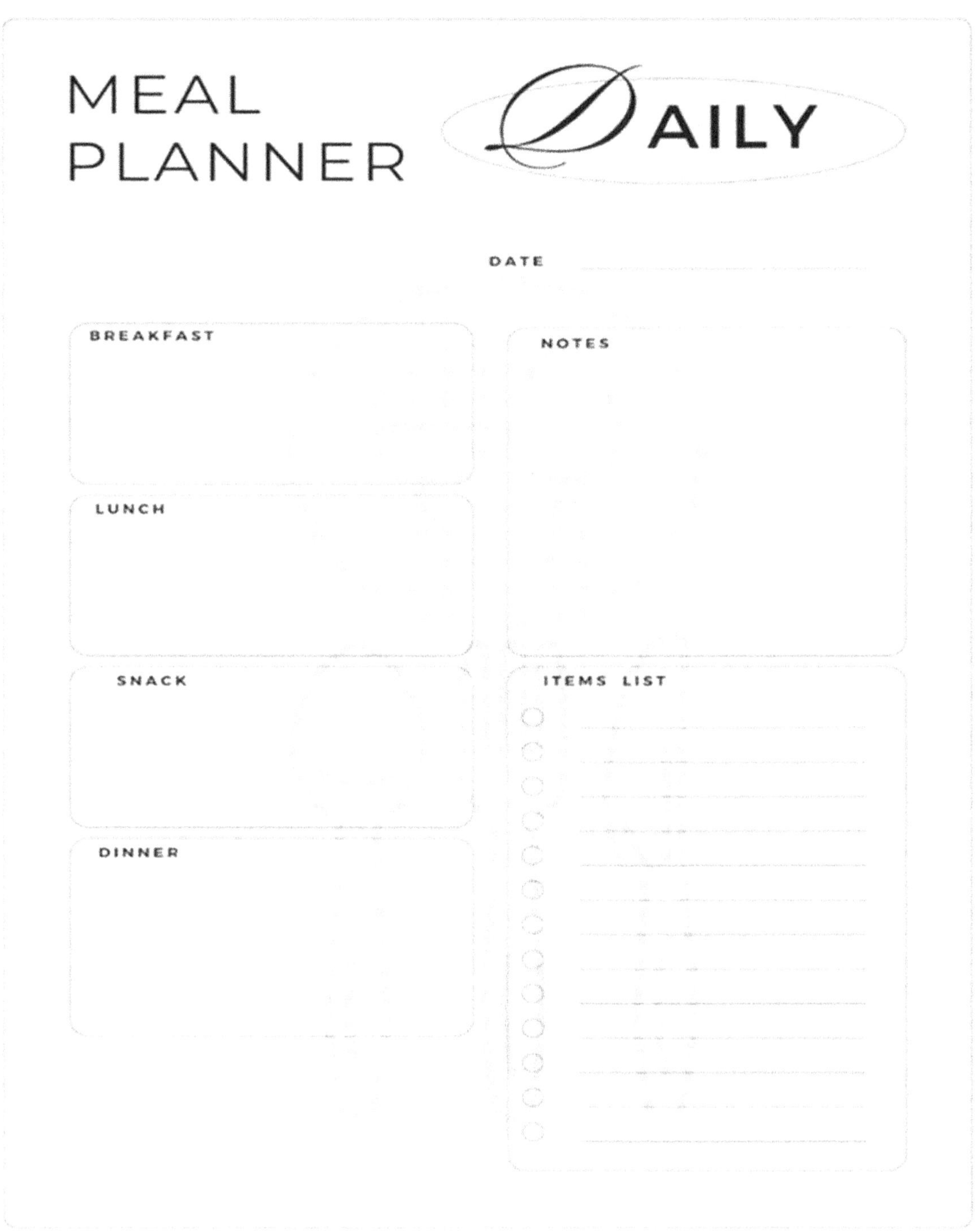

DAILY

DATE

BREAKFAST

NOTES

LUNCH

SNACK

ITEMS LIST

DINNER

MEAL PLANNER

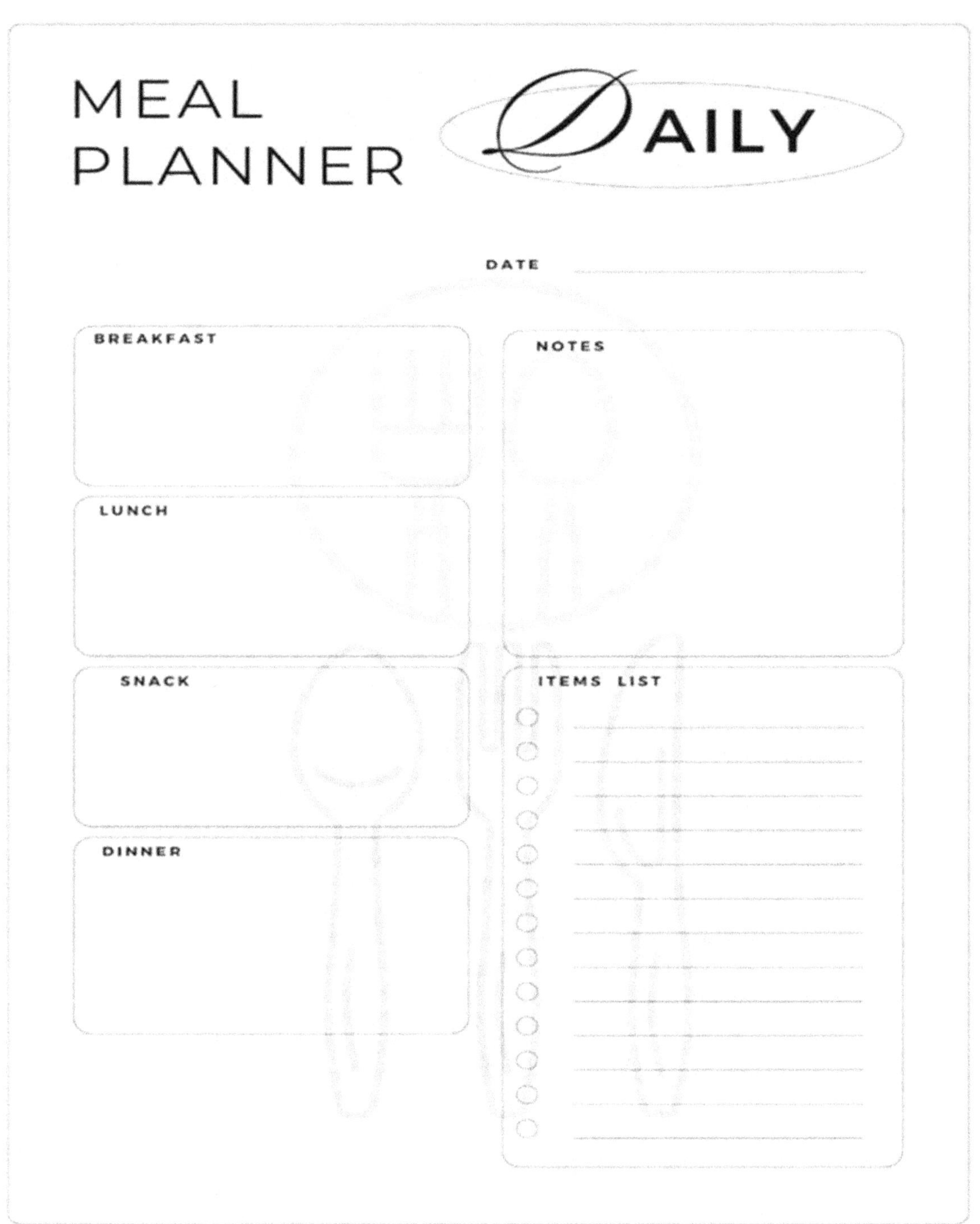

DAILY

DATE

BREAKFAST

NOTES

LUNCH

SNACK

ITEMS LIST

DINNER

MEAL PLANNER

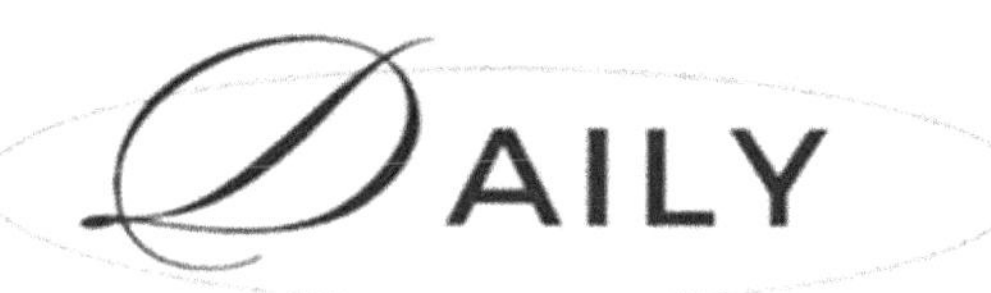

DATE

BREAKFAST

LUNCH

SNACK

DINNER

NOTES

ITEMS LIST